Blueprints

Clinical Cases in Family Medicine

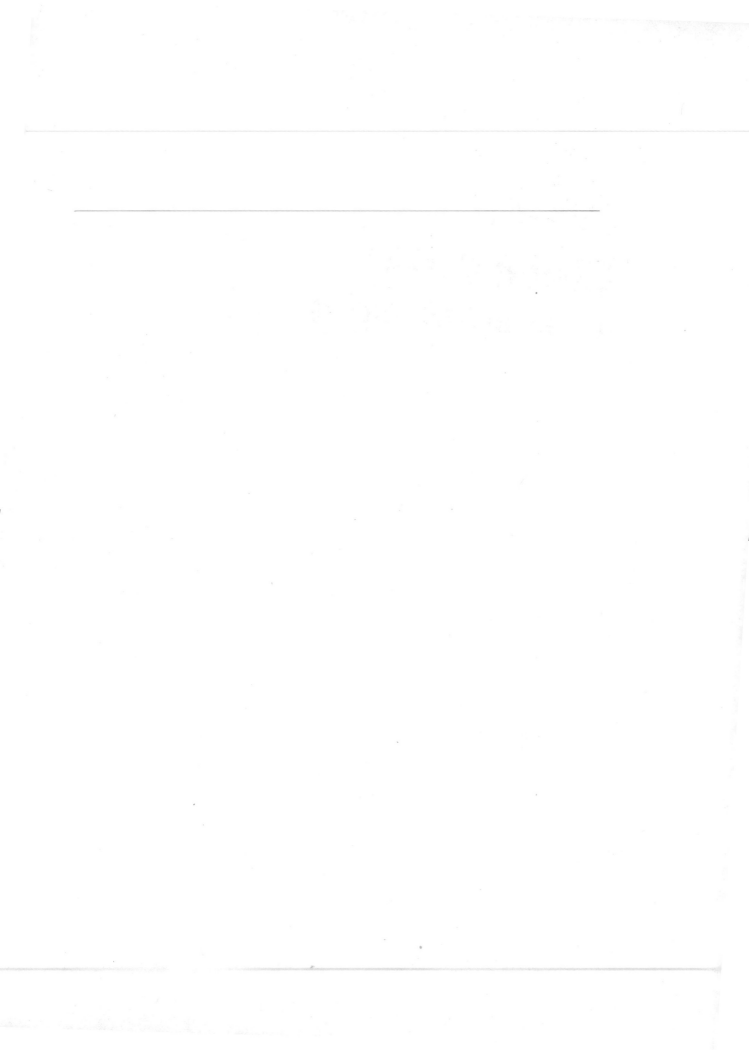

Blueprints
Clinical Cases in Family Medicine

Sarah Ellen Lesko, MD
  Family Physician
  San Francisco, California

Clea James, MD
  Private Practice Family Physician
  Columbia, South Carolina

Kimberly S. G. Chang, MD
  Resident Physician
  San Francisco General Hospital
  University of California, San Francisco
  San Francisco, California

Aaron B. Caughey, MD, MPP, MPH (Series Editor)
  Clinical Instructor, Division of Perinatology
  Department of Obstetrics & Gynecology
  University of California, San Francisco
  San Francisco, California

Blackwell
Publishing

© 2002 by Blackwell Science
a Blackwell Publishing Company

Blackwell Publishing, Inc., 350 Main Street, Malden, Massachusetts 02148-5018, USA
Blackwell Science Ltd., Osney Mead, Oxford OX2 0EL, UK
Blackwell Science Asia Pty Ltd, 550 Swanston Street, Carlton, Victoria 3053, Australia
Blackwell Verlag GmbH, Kurfürstendamm 57, 10707 Berlin, Germany

02 03 04 05 5 4 3 2 1

ISBN: 0-632-04654-6

Library of Congress Cataloging-in-Publication Data

Blueprints clinical cases in family medicine / by Sarah Ellen Lesko ... [et al.].
    p. ; cm. — (Blueprints clinical cases)
  ISBN 0-632-04654-6
  1. Family medicine. 2. Family medicine—Problems, exercises, etc.
  [DNLM: 1. Family Practice—Case Report. 2. Family Practice—Problems and Exercises.
WB 18.2 B6572 2002] I. Title: Clinical cases in family medicine. II. Lesko, Sarah Ellen.
III. Series.
  RA418.5.F3 B584 2002
  610'.76–dc21   2002007338

A catalogue record for this title is available from the British Library

Acquisitions: Beverly Copland
Development: Angela Gagliano
Production: Jennifer Kowalewski
Cover design: Hannus Designs
Interior design: Julie Gallagher
Typesetter: International Typesetting and Composition, in India
Printed and bound by Capital City Press, in Vermont

For further information on Blackwell Publishing, visit our website:
www.blackwellscience.com

Notice: The indications and dosages of all drugs in this book have been recommended in the medical literature and conform to the practices of the general community. The medications described and treatment prescriptions suggested do not
necessarily have specific approval by the Food and Drug Administration for use in
the diseases and dosages for which they are recommended. The package insert for
each drug should be consulted for use and dosage as approved by the FDA. Because
standards for usage change, it is advisable to keep abreast of revised recommendations, particularly those concerning new drugs.

DEDICATION

To my magnificent boys, Risley and Dylan, who have heard what actually happens if you jump on the bed while brushing your teeth; my captivating husband, Bob, who never complains when I tell gross stories at the dinner table; and my dear friends Beth and Ellen, who have taught me how to be a doctor.

Thank You!
Sarah Lesko

I dedicate this book to all the hardworking obstetrics residents at Valley Medical Center in San Jose, California. They saw me writing these cases in between messy deliveries on endless night calls, so that my few hours out of the hospital could be spent with my baby, Sebastian. Their humor, friendship, and compassion despite lack of sleep and nutrition sustained me through a difficult year and emphasized to me the importance of maintaining dignity and grace, no matter what the situation.

With best wishes for happiness and adventure to you all,
Clea James

*This is dedicated to God and angels for love and miracles that happen every day, whether we realize it or not. For my late grandfather, John K. H. Yee, and my grandmother Gladys Yee; my parents T. Irving and Jocelyn Chang; my siblings, Timothy, Allison, Jonathan, and Gina Chang; and for the incredible people at the UCSF-SFGH Family Practice Residency Program, especially the patients and my fellow residents, who have taught me an enormous amount about healing, faith, and love: Amy Kustra, MD, Stephanie Tache, MD, MPH, and Deborah Borne, MD, MSW—you **ROCK!** My special thanks go to Arthur D. Fu, MD, and Ray Hsu, MD, for their pictorial contributions that have greatly enhanced this book.*

Kimberly S. G. Chang

Thank you to Sarah, Clea, and Kim for outstanding work on this book, as well as all of the hardworking people at Blackwell Publishing, in particular Bev Copland, Angela Gagliano, and Jen Kowalewski. I would also like to thank Jim and Wendy, Pat and Kellie, Hennessey and Richard, Mike and Anda, Alisa and Jon, Tim and Kristen, Mike and Aoy, Kathy and Farouc, Deirdre and Max for each being such important parts of my life. Finally, I thank Susan and her family, Lieu, Ngan, Michael, Vivian, Robert, Kim, Mike, Nancy, Elizabeth, Winnie, and Sabrina, who will soon be my family, too.

Aaron

CONTENTS

CONTENTS

PREFACE

Medical education, a time-intensive process (as you know!), follows a largely predictable course. Along that path, the education becomes more inspiring as contact with actual patients increases. Learning medicine patient by patient is much more exhilarating than the heavy textbooks and endless slides of college science classes and the first two years of medical school. By now you are discovering the intensity of learning about disease processes simultaneously as your patients experience them. Along with this heightened learning environment comes a more stressful training situation, as attending physicians quiz you on morning rounds, patients urgently question you about their diagnoses and treatments, and you are expected to take in-service and Board examinations. We hope that these clinical case scenarios help you to refine your medical thinking process, focus on the relevant diseases and treatment modalities, improve your patient communication skills, and enable you to do well on the required examinations.

Through these cases we also hope that you will experience the rigors, challenges, and great satisfaction of family practice. The *Blueprints Clinical Cases* series has been designed to aid in preparation for medical school clinical rotations and in-service and Board examinations. *Blueprints Clinical Cases in Family Medicine* has been written to represent the family practice specialty, and therefore incorporates many major disease processes and organ systems, inpatient and outpatient medicine, adult and pediatric patients, male and female patients, acute and chronic conditions, and established as well as brand-new patients. The discipline of family practice focuses on the patients in the context of their daily lives, taking into account their family history, their jobs, their relationships, their personalities, and their life experiences.

Working through each case is similar to seeing the patients in person. During an actual patient visit, as you walk into the exam room you see only the Chief Complaint on the chart. After you introduce yourself, the patient relates the History of Present Illness; during each sentence you are formulating a differential diagnosis in your mind. As you ask about the Past Medical History, Past Surgical History, Family History, and current Medications, you hone down this differential diagnosis list, and then proceed to the physical exam and possibly further diagnostic testing. The case formats are designed to mimic the actual patient encounter, and the Thought Questions sprinkled throughout each case are designed to mimic your thought processes as you interact with the patient. Although during an actual patient visit the process of formulating and narrowing down the differential diagnosis necessarily occurs quickly, please take time to fully address each Thought Question, writing down possible answers in the margin and practicing your medical decision skills. In the interest of space, only the pertinent positive and negative findings are mentioned in the cases, although you will not find this to be true in actual patient encounters! The multiple-choice questions and answers at the end of the cases are designed to expand your knowledge about the case subject.

We hope this case book helps further your medical education and gives you a sense of the rewards and challenges of family practice. Good luck—remember to enjoy the process.

Sarah Ellen Lesko
Clea James
Kimberly S. G. Chang
Aaron B. Caughey

ABBREVIATIONS/ACRONYMS

%ile	percentile
##% RA	##% oxygen saturation on room air
AAA	abdominal aortic aneurysm
AAFP	American Academy of Family Physicians
AAP	American Academy of Pediatricians
ACIP	American Committee on Infectious Diseases
Ab	antibody
ABCs	airway, breathing, circulation assessment
Abd	abdomen
ABGs	arterial blood gases
ACE	angiotensin-converting enzyme
ACL	anterior cruciate ligament of the knee
ADHD	attention-deficit hyperactivity disorder
ADLs	activities of daily living
AFDC	Aid to Families with Dependent Children
AFP	alpha fetoprotein
AHA	American Heart Association
AI	aortic insufficiency
AIDS	acquired immunodeficiency syndrome
ALL	allergies
ALT	alanine transaminase
AMA	against medical advice
ANA	antinuclear antibody
ARB	angiotensin receptor blocker
ARDS	adult respiratory distress syndrome
ARF	acute renal failure
AS	aortic stenosis
ASA	acetylsalicylic acid (aspirin)
ASCUS	abnormal squamous cells of unknown significance
AST	aspartate transaminase
ATN	acute tubular necrosis
AVM	arteriovenous malformation
BCC	basal cell carcinoma
BCG	bacillus Calmette-Guerin (vaccine against tuberculosis)
BCM	birth control method
bid	twice a day
BLQ	bilateral lower quadrant
BM	bowel movement
BME	bimanual exam
BMI	body mass index
BMP	basic metabolic panel
BP	blood pressure
BPH	benign prostatic hypertrophy
BRBPR	bright red blood per rectum
BS	bowel sounds
BUN	blood urea nitrogen
CA	cancer
CABG	coronary artery bypass graft
CAD	coronary artery disease
CBC	complete blood count
cc	cubic centimeter
C/C/E	cords, clubbing, or edema
CDC	Center for Disease Control
CHF	congestive heart failure

CIWA	Clinical Institute Withdrawal Assessmet for Alcohol
CK	creatine kinase
Cl⁻	chloride
CMT	cervical motion tenderness
CMV	cytomegalovirus
CN	cranial nerve(s)
CNS	central nervous system
CO	carbon monoxide
CO₂	carbon dioxide
Coags	see PT and PTT
COPD	chronic obstructive pulmonary disease
CP	chest pain
CPK	creatine phosphokinase
CR	creatinine
C&S	culture and sensitivities
C/S	Cesarean section
CSF	cerebrospinal fluid
CT	computed tomography
CTA	clear to auscultation
CV	cardiovascular
CVA	cerebrovascular accident
CVAT	costovertebral angle tenderness
CXR	chest x-ray
D	diarrhea
D&C	dilatation and curettage
DBP	diastolic blood pressure
DDx	differential diagnosis
DI	diabetes insipidus
DIC	disseminated intravascular coagulation
DJD	degenerative joint disease
DKA	diabetic ketoacidosis
DLCO	diffusing capacity of the lung for carbon monoxide
DM	diabetes mellitus
DM 2	diabetes mellitus type 2
DNA	deoxyribonucleic acid
DNR/DNI	do not resuscitate/do not intubate
DP	dorsalis pedis
DPOA	durable power of attorney
DRE	digital rectal exam
DT	delirium tremens
DTRs	deep tendon reflexes
DVT	deep venous thrombosis
E&C	electrodessication and curettage
ECG/EKG	electrocardiography
Echo	echocardiography
ED	emergency department
EF	ejection fraction
EG	external genitalia
EGD	esophagogastroduodenoscopy
EOMI	extraocular movements intact
ER	emergency room
ERCP	endoscopic retrograde cholangiopancreatography
ESR	erythrocyte sedimentation rate
ESRD	end stage renal disease

EtOH	ethanol
Ex-lap	exploratory laparotomy
Ext	extremities (physical examination)
F/C	fever/chills
$FeSO_4$	ferrous sulfate (iron)
FeNa	fractional excretion of sodium; $100 \times [(pCr \times uNa)/(uCr \times pNa)]$
FEV1	forced expiratory volume in 1 second
FH	fundal height
FHT	fetal heart tones
FHx	family history
FOBT	fecal occult blood test
FSBG	finger stick blood glucose
FT4	free T-4
g	gram
G#P#	pregnancy# live birth#
Ga.	gauge (needle width)
GA	gestational age
GC	gonococcus/gonorrhea
GEN	general appearance (physical exam)
GERD	gastroesophageal reflux disease
GFR	glomerular filtration rate
GGT	gamma glutamyl transferase
GI	gastrointestinal
Gluc	glucose
GM	grandmother
gtt	drops
GU	genitourinary
GYNHx	gynecologic history
H&P	history and physical
HA	headache
HCG	human chorionic gonadotropin
HBcAb	hepatitis B core antibody
HBeAg	hepatitis B early antigen
HBsAb	hepatitis B surface antibody
HBsAg	hepatitis B surface antigen
HBV	hepatitis B virus
HCO_3	bicarbonate
Hct	hematocrit
HCTZ	hydrochlorothiazide
HCV	hepatitis C virus
HDL	high density lipoprotein
HEENT	head, eyes, ears, nose, and throat
Hgb	hemoglobin
HgbA1c	glycosylated hemoglobin; averages 3 month blood sugar level
Hib	Hemophilus influenza type b
HIV	human immunodeficiency virus
HPI	history of present illness
HPV	human papilloma virus
HR	heart rate
HRT	hormone replacement therapy
HSM	hepatosplenomegaly
Ht	height
HTN	hypertension
HSV	herpes simplex virus
IADLs	instrumental activities of daily living
IBD	inflammatory bowel disease
ICU	intensive care unit
ID	infectious disease
ID/CC	identification and chief complaint
IDDM	insulin-dependent diabetes mellitus
I/E	inspiratory to expiratory ratio
Ig	immunoglobulin
IM	intramuscular
IMM	immunization
INH	isoniazid
INR	international normalized ratio (standardized PT)
IUD	intrauterine device
IUGR	intrauterine growth restriction/retardation
IUP	intrauterine pregnancy
IV	intravenous
IVF	intravenous fluids
IVDU	intravenous drug use
IVP	intravenous pyelogram
IVIG	intravenous immunoglobulin
JVD	jugular venous distention
JVP	jugular venous pressure
K	potassium
KS	Kaposi's sarcoma
KUB	kidneys/ureter/bladder
LAN/LAD	lymphadenopathy
LBBB	left bundle-branch block
LDH	lactate dehydrogenase
LDL	low-density lipoprotein
LE	lower extremities
LES	lower esophageal sphincter
LFTs	liver function tests
LGSIL	low-grade squamous intra-epithelial lesion
LHRH	luteinizing hormone releasing hormone
LLE	left lower extremity
LMN	lower motor neuron
LMP	last menstrual period
LMWH	low molecular weight heparin
LP	lumbar puncture
LSB	left sternal border
LTBI	latent tuberculosis infection
LV	left ventricular
LVH	left ventricular hypertrophy
MAOI	monoamine oxidase inhibitors
mcg	microgram
MCV	mean corpuscular volume
MDI	metered-dose inhaler
MEDS	medications
mg	milligram
MI	myocardial infarction
MJ	marijuana
MM	malignant melanoma
MMM	mucous membranes moist
MMR	measles mumps rubella vaccine
MR(I)	magnetic resonance (imaging)
MR	mitral regurgitation
M/R/G	murmur/rub/gallop
MVI	multivitamin
N	nausea
Na	sodium
NABS	normoactive bowel sounds
NAD	no acute distress
NC/AT	normocephalic/atraumatic
NCEP	national cholesterol education project
ND	non-distended (abdomen)
Neuro	neurologic physical examination
NG	nasogastric
NI	nonimmune
NIDDM	noninsulin-dependent diabetes mellitus
NIH	National Institutes of Health
NKDA	no known drug allergies
Nl	normal
NPO	nil per os (nothing by mouth)
NS	night sweats

ABBREVIATIONS/ACRONYMS

NSAID	nonsteroidal anti-inflammatory drug	RUQ	right upper quadrant
NSR	normal sinus rhythm	RV	right ventricular
NSVD	normal spontaneous vaginal delivery	RVH	right ventricular hypertrophy
NT	nontender (abdomen)	Rx	treatment or therapy
NTD	neural tube defect	S1,S2,S3,S4	1st, 2nd, 3rd, 4th heart sounds
NTG	nitroglycerine	SAB	spontaneous abortion
N/V	nausea/vomiting	SAH	subarachnoid hemorrhage
OBHx	obstetrical history	SaO$_2$	oxygen saturation
OCD	obsessive compulsive disorder	SBO	small bowel obstruction
OCPs	oral contraceptive pills	SBP	systolic blood pressure
OD	overdose	SCC	squamous cell carcinoma
OG	orogastric	SE	side effects
OP	oropharynx	SH	social history
OTC	over the counter	SLE	systemic lupus erythematosus
Ou	both eyes	SOB	shortness of breath
P	pulse	s/p	status post (event in past)
PAP	prostate acid phosphatase	SQ	subcutaneous
PCN	penicillin	SSE	sterile speculum exam
pCO$_2$	partial pressure of carbon dioxide	SSRI	selective serotonin reuptake inhibitor
PE	physical exam	ST	sinus tachycardia
PE	pulmonary embolism	STD	sexually transmitted disease
PERRLA	pupils equal, round and reactive to light and accommodation	Sxs	symptoms
		S/NT/ND	soft, nontender, nondistended (abdomen)
PFTs	pulmonary function tests		
pH	acid-base status	T	temperature
PID	pelvic inflammatory disease	TAB	therapeutic abortion
Plt	platelets	TB	tuberculosis
PMD	primary medical doctor	TCA	trichloroacetic acid
PMI	point of maximal impulse	TCA	tricyclic antidepressants
PMN	polymorphonuclear leukocyte	TFTs	thyroid function tests
PMHx/PSHx	past medical history/past surgical history	TG	triglyceride
PNL	prenatal labs	TIA	transient ischemic attack
PNV	prenatal vitamins	TIBC	total iron-binding capacity
po	per os (per mouth)	tid	three times a day
pO$_2$	partial pressure of oxygen	TM	tympanic membrane(s)
ppd	pack per day	TMJ	temporomandibular joint
PPD	purified protein derivative (test for tuberculosis)	TOA	tubo-ovarian abscess
		Tob	tobacco
PRN	as needed	TMP/SMX	trimethoprim/sulfamethoxazole
PSA	prostate-specific antigen	T&S	type and screen
PT	prothrombin time	TSH	thyroid-stimulating hormone
PTCA	percutaneous transluminal coronary angioplasty	TTP	tenderness to palpation
		UA	urinalysis
PTSD	post-traumatic stress disorder	Udip	dipstick urinalysis
PTT	partial thromboplastin time	UGI	upper GI
PUD	peptic ulcer disease	UMN	upper motor neuron
PVC	premature ventricular contraction	Uosm	urinary osmolality
Q # h	every # hours	URI	upper respiratory tract infection
qd	once a day	UTD	up-to-date
qhs	once at bedtime	UTZ	ultrasound
qid	four times a day	UTI	urinary tract infection
RA	room air	V	vomiting
RBC	red blood cell	VBAC	vaginal birth after cesarean section
RCA	right coronary artery	VCUG	voiding cystourethrogram
RCT	randomized controlled trial	VDRL	Venereal Disease Research Laboratory
Rh	rhesus antigen	VLDL	very-low-density lipoprotein
RLE	right lower extremity	V/Q	ventilation/perfusion
RLL	right lower lobe	VS	vital signs
RML	right middle lobe	VSD	ventriculoseptal defect
RN	registered nurse	WBC	white blood cell
ROM	range of motion	WDWN	well-developed, well-nourished
ROS	review of systems	WNL	within normal limits
RPR	rapid plasma reagin	Wt	weight
RR	respiratory rate	XRT	radiation therapy
RRR	regular rate and rhythm	y.o.	-year-old

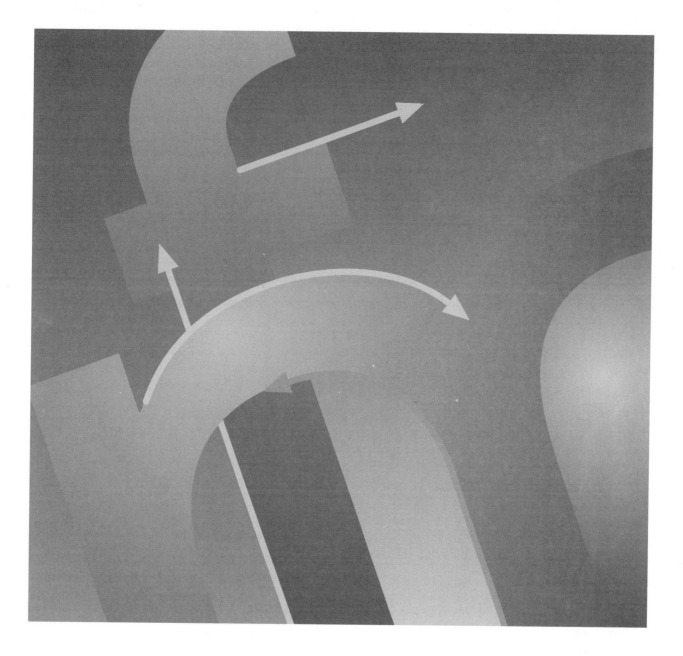

CASES

CASE **1** / **PRENATAL CARE**

ID/CC: PC is a 30-year-old G2P0 patient who presents to your office with a LMP eight weeks ago and a positive pregnancy test at home two days ago.

HPI: The patient stopped her birth control pills four months ago and this is a desired pregnancy. She comes in with lots of questions and hopes to establish prenatal care with you. She wants an ultrasound today as she had a little vaginal spotting this morning and is worried she will lose the pregnancy. Her last intercourse was last night. She wants to establish a birth plan and hopes to have no medications at all during her labor as she has been reading that even having an IV can impede the "natural birth process."

PMHx: Asthma, migraines   **PSHx:** None   **OBHx:** TAB two years ago at nine weeks

GYNHx: Normal Pap smears, regular periods, no STDs

Meds: Salmeterol inhaler twice a day, beclomethasone inhaler twice a day, Excedrin as needed

All: NKDA

FHx: Mother, sister, and maternal grandmother diabetes mellitus II, father myocardial infarction age 70

SHx: Tobacco 1/2 pack per day, no alcohol, no drug use

ROS: No cramping or contractions, nausea and vomiting once or twice each morning for the past week, some urinary frequency but no dysuria, no shortness of breath or chest pain, low back pain, heartburn occasionally

---

THOUGHT QUESTIONS
- What routine labs does this patient need?
- What other tests are standard of care?
- Does she need an ultrasound now?
- Are there any other tests you should consider?
- What kind of ultrasound should you order?

Routine prenatal care includes:

Initial OB visit:
   Labs: CBC, T&S, Rubella Ab, VDRL, urinalysis, HBsAg, GC, chlamydia
   Exam: BP, urine for glucose and protein, BME assessing uterine size, Pap smear
   Listen for FHT (won't hear if GA < 9–11 weeks)
   Consider: HIV, PPD

Every visit:
   BP, fundal height, FHT, urine dip for protein and glucose, ROS

15–20 weeks:
   triple screen, consider anatomic survey or dating ultrasound

28 weeks
   one-hour glucola, RhoGAM if Rh-negative

Routine gestational diabetes mellitus (GDM) screening is done at 28 weeks. However, in this patient with a positive family history of DM a one-hour glucola should be ordered as part of her routine prenatal labs now. Screening consists of a 50-gram glucola drink followed by a blood glucose measurement an hour later. An abnormal value is above 140. Other patients who need a glucola at the first prenatal care visit include women with glucosuria, a previous history of GDM, or a previous macrosomic or stillborn infant.

Unless she has continued vaginal bleeding or size ≠ dates on today's exam there is no need for an ultrasound at this time. The RADIUS trial (1993) suggested that routine screening ultrasound did not improve perinatal or maternal management or outcomes as compared with the selective use of ultrasound on the basis of clinician judgment.

The American Institute of Ultrasound in Medicine (AIUM) classifies obstetric ultrasound as either level I (Basic) or II (High Risk). A level I ultrasound can be done in any trimester, but a level II ultrasound targeting high-risk pregnancies is best performed in the second (or third) trimester.

Level I ultrasounds must document the following:
first trimester: location of gestational sac
                number of fetuses
                crown-rump length
                cardiac activity
                evaluation of uterus and adnexae
second and third trimester: fetal life
                number of fetuses
                presentation
                amniotic fluid volume
                placental location
                gestational age: composite of measurements from BPD
                    (biparietal diameter), HC (head circumference), AC
                    (abdominal circumference), and FL (femur length)
                basic fetal anatomy: cerebral ventricles, spine, stomach,
                    bladder, umbilical cord insertion site, kidneys,
                    four-chamber heart

Level II ultrasounds include the level I guidelines plus expanded criteria depending on the reason for the high-risk assessment; for example, BPP (biophysical profile), umbilical cord structure and function, placental morphology, detailed fetal morphology, and umbilical artery and middle cerebral artery blood flow and velocity waveforms.

VS: HR 84 BP 120/72 Weight 152 lbs

PE: Pleasant woman NAD. *Lungs:* CTA, CV RRR with soft holosystolic murmur no radiation. *Abdomen:* soft, nontender, fundus not palpable. *Extremities:* no edema. *Spec exam:* nulliparous os, no lesions seen, physiologic d/c. *BME:* anteverted midline uterus, about six-week size, no adnexal masses

Labs: O+, Ab–, VDRL NR, HBsAg–, Rubella NI, Hct 31, Pap WNL, GC and chlamydia negative, PPD negative, HIV negative, one-hour glucola 130, urine protein trace, glucose negative

QUESTIONS

1. The patient agrees to cut down on her smoking but says she can't quit cold turkey. What risks is smoking in pregnancy NOT associated with?
   A. Placental abruption
   B. Preterm birth
   C. Gestational diabetes
   D. Low birth weight

2. Her one-hour glucola is WNL with a cutoff of 140 being the standard. When should she have another glucose test checked?
   A. In four weeks
   B. At 28 weeks
   C. Only if she has glucosuria
   D. No need to check another one during this pregnancy

3. She asks about the "triple screen." You explain that it is a blood test of three hormones and helps predict the risk for all of the following EXCEPT:
   A. Neural tube defects
   B. Down syndrome
   C. Gastroschisis
   D. Sickle cell disease

4. A patient presents to your office and is trying to conceive. She is not currently taking prenatal vitamins. Why should you prescribe them for her now prior to her pregnancy?
   A. To reduce the risk for Down syndrome
   B. To reduce the risk for NTDs (neural tube defects)
   C. To decrease the risk for miscarriage
   D. To decrease the rate of hyperemesis in pregnancy

CASE 2 / PREGNANCY AND HYPERTENSION

ID/CC: PH is a 21-year-old G1P0 at 34 weeks gestational age who comes into your office for a routine OB check.

HPI: She has just moved from another state and did not bring her prior prenatal records with her, but denies any problems with the pregnancy so far. On glancing at the chart as you walk into the room you notice her BP is 142/85. She has a mild headache and complains of lower extremity edema for one week. She had some heartburn this past week with occasional nausea and vomiting. She denies any blurry vision, back pain, or dysuria. The baby moves well and she has not felt any contractions.

PMHx: None   **PSHx:** None   **Meds:** Prenatal vitamins, iron   **All:** NKDA

SHx: No smoking, one to two beers a week, no drugs. She works at a video store and lives with her boyfriend.

ROS: As above

THOUGHT QUESTIONS

- Is her BP significant?
- What questions do you want to ask?
- What is the differential diagnosis of elevated blood pressure in pregnancy?
- What will you focus on with PE and labs?

Elevated blood pressures always merit workup during pregnancy. The differential diagnosis includes 1) preeclampsia, 2) pregnancy-induced hypertension (PIH), and 3) chronic hypertension with or without exacerbation during pregnancy.

Preeclampsia includes the triad of hypertension (>140 SBP or >90 DBP), non-dependent edema, and proteinuria (>300 mg in 24 hours) after 20 weeks gestational age. It is more common in nulliparous patients, the extremes of reproductive age, chronic hypertension, DM, FHx preeclampsia, prior history of preeclampsia, and multiple gestations.

Pregnancy-induced hypertension is defined as elevated blood pressures after 20 weeks gestational age in the absence of proteinuria or pathologic edema. Often it is unclear whether this occurs in the setting of undiagnosed chronic hypertension vs. it truly being related to the pregnancy. Because both types of patients can be seen in this population, it is more common in women with a family history of hypertension and can predict hypertension later on in life. Elevated blood pressures before 20 weeks gestational age are almost always associated with chronic hypertension. Those patients are at a 15–25% increased risk for preeclampsia or pregnancy-associated hypertension later on in pregnancy.

Although this patient denies a prior history of hypertension and is only 21 years old, it would be helpful to get her old prenatal records and ensure her BPs were previously normal. An initial or "booking" blood pressure that is normal in the first trimester, supports a pregnancy-related issue. However, a normal blood pressure in the second trimester is of little help, as the blood pressure has already reached its nadir at this point in pregnancy. You should ask about classic preeclampsia symptoms such as headache, edema, epigastric pain, and blurred vision, and check her urine for protein.

CASE CONTINUED

VS: BP 142/85 sitting, 138/78 lying down, 154/92 standing up

PE: NAD, lungs CTA, CV RRR, FH 34 cm, FHT 140s. Extremities 2+ edema LE, 1+ edema hands, DTRs 2+ with 1-beat clonus. *Urine dip:* protein 2+, glucose negative

4

Her H&P and proteinuria are consistent with preeclampsia. You send the patient over to the hospital for further evaluation and ask for the following labs: CBC, chem-7, uric acid, AST, catheterized urinalysis.

Labs: Platelets 125, Hct 41, Uric Acid 8.5, Creatinine 0.8, AST 39

Catheterized urinalysis: 1+ protein

THOUGHT QUESTIONS
- What causes preeclampsia?
- What is the treatment?
- What do the labs mean?

Preeclampsia is the result of reduced organ perfusion caused by vasospasm of unclear etiology. When the vasospasm is severe the patient can have hepatocellular necrosis, hemolysis, platelet aggregation and activation, cerebral and neurologic symptoms, and even worsening proteinuria and renal ischemia with resultant oliguria, pulmonary edema, seizures, and stroke.

The most commonly involved organ systems include the kidneys, liver, and hematologic system. In the kidneys, vasospasm leads to a reduction in GFR, often resulting in increased serum uric acid levels, proteinuria, and in severe cases increasing creatinine levels. In the liver, elevations of serum transaminases can be seen, and in extremely rare cases hepatic rupture can occur, which carries a maternal mortality rate of 70%.

Vasospasm and disruption of the vascular endothelium can lead to thrombocytopenia. Hemolysis is also a result, and probably comes from RBCs passing through small blood vessels with damaged intima and fibrin deposition. Hemolysis can be documented by an abnormal peripheral smear, decreasing hematocrit, increased total bilirubin, or increased LDH (>600 U/L). In preeclampsia hemolysis is defined as the presence of a microangiopathic hemolytic anemia, and is the hallmark of HELLP syndrome (hemolysis, elevated liver enzymes, low platelets). HELLP complicates less than 10% of cases of severe preeclampsia.

Of all complications of preeclampsia, eclampsia (seizure activity) may be the most dreaded. The mechanism of eclampsia is largely unclear, and may be only partially associated with hypertension and vascular spasm. In fact, 20% of eclamptic patients have no preceding proteinuria or headache.

The definitive treatment for preeclampsia is delivery. Although much research has been devoted to finding prophylactic treatments for preeclampsia, nothing has been found to prevent or cure preeclampsia other than delivery of the fetus.

QUESTIONS

5. You order a 24-hour urine for protein to decide whether her preeclampsia is mild or severe. Criteria that would establish a diagnosis of severe preeclampsia in this patient include:
   A. BP > 150/90
   B. Uric acid elevation
   C. Severe headache
   D. Platelets 125,000

6. Complications of preeclampsia include all the following EXCEPT:
   A. Eclampsia
   B. Abruption
   C. IUGR
   D. Severe anemia

7. You decide to induce the patient. Along with your induction agent you give the patient
   A. Nifedipine to control her blood pressure
   B. Magnesium for seizure prophylaxis
   C. Demerol for her headache
   D. IVF open-wide to treat her volume depletion

8. If this were a patient with chronic hypertension, what medication would you use for blood pressure control?
   A. Labetalol
   B. Lisinopril
   C. Magnesium
   D. All blood pressure medication is contraindicated during pregnancy

ID/CC: SB is a 34-year-old G2P2 who presents to the ER with a one-day history of vaginal bleeding and pelvic cramping. Her LMP was nine weeks ago.

HPI: The patient denies any recent illnesses and states that her periods are somewhat irregular. The cramping is more severe than period pains and is worsening over the course of the day. She denies dysuria but does complain of low back pain and urinary frequency. She has had some white vaginal discharge recently. The bleeding started lightly and now is a little heavier. She used two pads today and denies passing any clots or products of conception.

PMHx: None   **PSHx:** Lumbar spine surgery two years ago   **Meds:** Acetaminophen as needed

All: NKDA   **GYNHx:** Chlamydia age 24 and again age 31, no Pap smear since her last pregnancy

OBHx: NSVD x 2   **BCM:** IUD, placed after her last delivery four years ago

FHx: Sister and mother have both had one SAB and two full-term pregnancies each, no multiple gestations, aneuploidy, or stillbirths

---

THOUGHT QUESTIONS

- What is the next thing you want to know?
- What is the differential diagnosis and what risk factors does the patient have?

After ascertaining that the patient has stable VS, a pregnancy test is essential. The differential diagnosis includes a threatened abortion, an ectopic pregnancy, cervical lesions, trophoblastic disorders, or menometrorrhagia. Risk factors for an ectopic pregnancy in this patient include IUD use and prior history of chlamydia. Other risk factors for ectopic pregnancies include prior tubal ligation, other pelvic surgeries, PID (pelvic inflammatory disease), IVF (in vitro fertilization), or diethylstilbestrol (DES) exposure. Abdominal pain (94% of women with ectopic pregnancies) and irregular vaginal bleeding (80%) are the most common presenting symptoms in ectopic pregnancy. Only one-half of patients with an ectopic pregnancy have a palpable abdominal mass.

VS: Temp. 98.2°F BP 102/68 HR 100 RR 18

PE: WDWN woman NAD. Lungs CTA, CV RRR. Abdomen soft with BLQ mild tenderness without rebound or guarding. BME: slightly enlarged uterus that is midline and mildly tender, mild right adnexal tenderness without mass appreciated, os closed with some blood in the vault, no lesions on the cervix

Labs: Urine βhCG positive, Hct 37, serum βhCG 2200 mIU

THOUGHT QUESTION

- The patient sits in the ER crying, sure that she will have a miscarriage because of her family history of SABs. You explain to the patient that about 30% of all pregnancies end in spontaneous abortion and therefore the odds are possible that she will have a SAB but probably not related to family history. What are the risk factors and workup for *recurrent* spontaneous abortions?

Recurrent SAB is defined as the loss of more than three pregnancies before 20 weeks gestational age, and applies to about 0.3% of pregnant women. The risk for a miscarriage is 15% after one loss, 24% after two losses, 30% after three losses, and 40% after four consecutive losses.

The causes for SAB in general include an anembryonic gestation (blighted ovum), embryonic anomalies, chromosomal anomalies (26% of all losses are due to trisomy 16), advanced maternal age, uterine anomalies, IUD in place, teratogen exposure, mutagen exposure, maternal disease, placental anomalies, and extensive maternal trauma.

The causes for recurrent SAB include chromosomal anomalies, autoimmune disorders (especially lupus anticoagulant and antiphospholipid syndrome), endocrine disease (thyroid, diabetes, prolactin, androgen disorders, luteal phase disorders), infections (bacteria, viruses, parasites, fungi), and uterine anomalies (incompetent cervix, leiomyomas, etc.). Of all the causes chromosomal anomalies comprise 60% of cases, and women over age 35 have an eight to 10 times higher risk of a chromosomal etiology to their recurrent SABs.

Work up patients with recurrent SABs by evaluating a thorough history of both partners, family histories, careful physical exam, and consider the following labs: parental and abortal karyotypes, TSH, lupus anticoagulant, anticardiolipin antibody, CBC, endometrial biopsy during the luteal phase, and an intrauterine cavity assessment using hysteroscopy or a hysterosalpingogram.

Although many doctors try to treat threatened SABs with bed rest, oral or intravaginal progesterone, or sedatives, there is no evidence of any effective treatment. Studies have also been performed trying to treat women with a history of recurrent SAB using steroids, low-dose aspirin, heparin, or intravenous Ig, but the results are inconclusive so far.

You are concerned about an ectopic pregnancy and order a TVUS (transvaginal ultrasound).

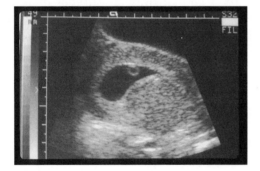

FIGURE 3 An early intrauterine pregnancy with a yolk sac. (Image provided by Departments of Radiology and Obstetrics & Gynecology, University of California, San Francisco.)

QUESTIONS

9. What do you expect to see if she has an IUP (intrauterine pregnancy)?
   A. Too early to see anything in uterus
   B. Gestational sac
   C. Fetus with cardiac motion
   D. A trans-abdominal ultrasound is more sensitive to see an IUP

10. If the ultrasound is equivocal and the patient is stable another option is serial serum βhCG. Which statement is correct?
   A. The normal doubling time for hCG is 96h
   B. One-third of ectopics have a normal doubling time
   C. An abnormal serial hCG is diagnostic of an ectopic pregnancy
   D. βhCG is only useful when compared to serum progesterone levels

11. Treatment alternatives for ectopic pregnancy include:
   A. Surgical excision
   B. Cyclophosphamide
   C. D&C
   D. No need to treat until the ectopic ruptures

12. In your patient the ultrasound shows no adnexal masses and a gestational sac with IUP in the uterus. You diagnose the patient with a:
   A. Threatened abortion
   B. Inevitable abortion
   C. Incomplete abortion
   D. Missed abortion

ID/CC: IN is your last patient of the day, and you are admitting her for induction.

HPI: This is a 27-year-old G1P0 at 42 weeks by LMP and 30-week ultrasound. Her pregnancy has been uncomplicated. She feels irregular contractions without vaginal bleeding or loss of fluid. The baby is moving well. She has had reactive NSTs (non-stress tests) twice weekly since 40 weeks gestational age.

PMHx: None   **PSHx:** Appendectomy age 14   **OBHx:** Nullipara

Meds: Prenatal vitamins, iron   **All:** NKDA

THOUGHT QUESTIONS

- What are some criteria for induction of labor?
- What are the risks of postdates pregnancy?
- When is antepartum testing recommended and what does it include?

Induction of labor should be considered for preeclampsia, premature rupture of membranes, chorioamnionitis, suspected fetal jeopardy (severe IUGR [intrauterine growth retardation], isoimmunization, etc.), maternal medical problems (DM, renal failure, COPD, etc.), IUFD (intrauterine fetal demise), and postdates pregnancy. Any pregnancy continuing past 42 weeks is considered postdates.

Risks of a postdates pregnancy include fetal macrosomia and resultant cephalopelvic disproportion, IUFD, meconium aspiration syndrome, and fetal birth trauma from macrosomia. Antepartum testing begins at 40 weeks and includes biweekly NSTs and AFIs (amniotic fluid index); a nonreactive NST necessitates a BPP (biophysical profile), and for an AFI less than five consider induction.

THOUGHT QUESTION

- What initial induction agent would be the best choice?

In a patient with a closed cervix, cervical ripening increases the chances of a successful induction and may decrease the risk for a cesarean section. Pharmacologic agents for cervical ripening include prostaglandin gel and prostaglandin tablets (misoprostol). Side effects include a 1–5% incidence of uterine hyperstimulation with possible effects on the FHT. These agents, especially misoprostol, are associated with higher rates of uterine rupture in patients with prior uterine scars (c-section, myomectomy) and therefore are relatively contraindicated in such patients. For these patients, cervical ripening can be achieved with mechanical agents such as Foley bulbs or laminaria inserted into the cervix. Mechanical agents can cause discomfort and bleeding, although they are usually tolerated very well. Mechanical and pharmacologic agents have been shown to have roughly equivalent efficacy.

CASE CONTINUED

VS: Temp 99.2°F BP 110/65 HR 100 RR 18

PE: Lungs CTA, CV RRR, Fundus 39 cm. *Vaginal exam:* cervix fingertip, 0% effaced, −2 station. EFW 3800 gm by Leopold's, vertex by ultrasound

The patient is admitted and given 25 micrograms of misoprostol intravaginally. After four hours you recheck and her cervical exam is 2 cm, 80% effaced, and −1 station.

THOUGHT QUESTIONS

- Is that latent or active phase?
- What stage of labor is it?

Labor is divided into three stages:

> stage 1: interval between onset of labor and full cervical dilation (10 cm)
> stage 2: interval between full cervical dilation and delivery of infant
> stage 3: interval between delivery of infant and delivery of placenta

Stage 1 is further divided into latent phase (closed cervix → <4 cm dilated) and active phase (4 cm → 10 cm dilated), also commonly considered to require frequent strong contractions).

The above definitions are not particularly relevant or necessary for normal labor that progresses well without problems, but do help identify abnormal labor patterns early on and assist the doctor to assess appropriate intervention to ensure a healthy baby and mom.

TABLE 4. Labor Patterns

STAGE	NULLIPARA MEAN/MAX	MULTIPARA MEAN/MAX
1	10 hours/<25 hours	8 hours/<19 hours
2	33 minutes/<2 hours	8 minutes/<46 minutes
3	5 minutes/<30 minutes	5 minutes/<30 minutes
latent phase	6 hours/<20 hours	5 hours/<14 hours
active phase	>1.2 cm dil. per hour	>1.5 cm dil. per hour

Abnormal patterns can be classified as prolonged vs. arrest. Appropriate interventions would include:

stage 1: prolonged latent phase: rest, Pitocin, pain medications; prolonged active phase: Pitocin, amniotomy, pain medications; active phase arrest: assess EFW, fetal station, presentation, position, clinical pelvimetry, IUPC to document adequate uterine activity. If indicated and more than two hours elapse: probable c-section

stage 2: arrest of descent: assess uterine contractility and cephalopelvic relationships, empty bladder; if station +2 try forceps or vacuum, otherwise probable c-section

QUESTIONS

13. After the cervix is ripened the patient is started on Pitocin IV. She does not feel strong contractions and you increase the dose every 30 minutes. Possible complications of Pitocin include all of the following EXCEPT:
    A. Uterine hyperstimulation
    B. Maternal hyponatremia
    C. Uterine rupture
    D. Pulmonary embolism

14. The patient would like an epidural but is worried it will affect her labor. Which statement is correct:
    A. It will approximately double the time of stage 1 of labor
    B. It will have no effect on stage 1, but cause a much higher risk for c-section
    C. A "walking epidural" has less effect on labor
    D. Side effects affect less than 10% of patients

15. Two hours later the nurse calls you because the patient is only contracting every 5 to 6 minutes. Her cervical exam is 5 cm dilation, 100% effacement, +1 station and you proceed with amniotomy for a diagnosis of:
    A. Prolonged active phase progress
    B. Arrest of dilation
    C. Arrest of descent
    D. Normal active phase progress

16. The patient becomes completely dilated and starts to push. 45 minutes into the second stage, the fetal heart tracing is as follows.

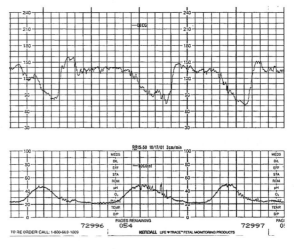

FIGURE 4 Fetal heart tracing.

The patient is bringing the head of the fetus down slightly with each push. You:
    A. Perform an emergent c-section
    B. Continue pushing with the patient
    C. Stop the Pitocin
    D. Give terbutaline for uterine hyperstimulation

CASE 5 / BREAST MASS

ID/CC: FB is a 41-year-old G0P0 who comes in for evaluation of a lump in her right breast.

HPI: The patient felt the lump last week and is very worried it could be cancer. Her sister had a lump removed many years ago, the patient thinks it might have been a "benign tumor." The patient has breast tenderness before her periods and has been told by past doctors that she has lumpy breasts, but this mass is new and concerning to the patient. The lump is somewhat tender. The patient has never had a mammogram.

The patient had some brownish discharge from her right breast two weeks ago. She has never had any discharge before, and denies any history of blood in the discharge that appeared two weeks ago.

PMHx: None **PSHx:** None **OBHx:** Nulliparous

GYNHx: Regular periods, normal Paps, menarche age 13, 15 years of OCPs total

Meds: Motrin as needed **All:** NKDA **FHx:** No history of breast or ovarian cancer

---

THOUGHT QUESTIONS
- What is the differential diagnosis of a breast mass?
- What workup is indicated in this patient?
- What risk factors does she have for breast cancer?

The differential diagnosis of a breast mass includes breast cancer, a cyst, a fibroadenoma, or fat necrosis. Although a breast mass is the most common presentation of breast cancer, 90% of breast masses are caused by benign lesions. In order to rule out breast cancer, you need to perform a careful physical exam, and based on your findings decide whether a mammogram, ultrasound, and/or biopsy is warranted. Risk factors for breast cancer include increasing age, family history, nulliparity or first delivery over age 30, obesity, menarche before age 12, menopause after age 50, or a history of ionizing radiation. The use of hormone replacement therapy may increase the risk slightly.

THOUGHT QUESTION
- What imaging studies are useful for evaluating a breast mass?

The most commonly used imagining modality is the mammogram. A slowly growing breast cancer can be seen on a mammogram more than two years before reaching a palpable size. Cancer typically appears as clustered pleomorphic microcalcifications, with a mammographic mass density with irregular or ill-defined borders. The sensitivity of mammogram ranges from 60% to 90% and depends on age, breast density, breast size, and location of masses. The specificity is 30–40% for nonpalpable mammographic abnormalities, and 85–90% for palpable masses.

Indications for a mammogram include:

1) Annual screening for breast cancer: one-third of abnormal masses on mammogram are malignant on biopsy. Screening usually starts between 40 and 50 years of age.
2) Evaluate a breast mass found on PE.
3) Search for occult breast cancer in a patient with metastatic disease in axillary nodes or elsewhere from an unknown primary tumor.
4) Follow breast cancer patients who have been treated with breast-conserving surgery and/or radiation.

Other imaging options include ultrasound and MRI. Ultrasound is not helpful for breast cancer screening as it does not detect microcalcifications, and instead is usually employed to distinguish benign cysts from solid tumors, for which it has a 95–100% accuracy.

MRI has a very high sensitivity but a low specificity, resulting in biopsy of many benign lesions, and therefore is also not a good screening tool. MRI is good at helping distinguish between scar and recurrent tumor in women with a history of breast cancer, and also at distinguishing between inflammation and tumor in women with breast implants: it can screen for cancer or locate silicon released by ruptured implants.

THOUGHT QUESTION
- What are some causes of nipple discharge in nonlactating women?

The differential diagnosis of nipple discharge includes carcinoma, intraductal papilloma, and fibro-cystic change with ectasia of the ducts. Galactorrhea (usually bilateral) can be caused by a pro-lactinoma, hypothyroidism, and medications such as phenothiazines and birth control pills.

VS: Temp 98°F BP 147/86 HR 90

PE: Breast exam: bilateral breasts have normal-appearing skin without dimpling or nipple retraction, no masses are observed. On palpation, both breasts are indeed somewhat lumpy, however a firm 1 cm discrete mass is palpable in the upper outer quadrant of the right breast; it is firm, tender and some-what mobile. No nipple discharge, no axillary or supraclavicular lymphadenopathy.

On aspiration with an 18-Ga. needle, greenish liquid is removed and the mass completely disappears.

QUESTIONS

17. What PE findings are associated with breast cancer?
    A. Bilateral lumps
    B. Painful nodule
    C. Rubbery consistency
    D. Fixed to skin or muscle

18. On PE you diagnosed a possible cyst, which you successfully aspirated. What is your next step?
    A. Send the fluid for cytology stat
    B. Surgical biopsy at the cyst site
    C. Schedule for recheck in four to six weeks
    D. Mammogram

19. How would you proceed if you palpate a solid mass on future exams in this patient?
    A. Fine needle aspiration biopsy
    B. Annual mammograms
    C. Mastectomy
    D. Recheck in three to six months

20. At her next visit the patient has no complaints and PE is within normal limits. What screening recommendations are appropriate?
    A. Mammograms starting age 40
    B. Clinical breast exam and mammogram every other year
    C. Breast self-exam each month plus annual mammogram
    D. Annual clinical breast exam, mammograms starting age 50, breast self-exam up to patient discretion

CASE 6 / URINARY INCONTINENCE

ID/CC: SI is a 67-year-old woman who comes in for her routine annual physical. On ROS she complains of urinary incontinence.

HPI: The patient describes incontinence with coughing, laughing, and brisk exercise. She has begun wearing pads in her underwear and is vexed by her slowly worsening symptoms. She denies any dysuria. She urinates once during the night and five to six times during the day, although she estimates that she also involuntarily leaks urine two to three times a day. She never feels that she can't get to the bathroom in time to urinate. She drinks three to four glasses of water a day, a cup of coffee in the morning, and has recently cut out her evening coffee in the hopes that it would help her incontinence.

She is sexually active and has mild dyspareunia about half of the time; lubricants seem to help. She denies any history of pyelonephritis, although she has had two to three UTIs a year for the past five years. She notices that the incontinence is worse when her COPD is acting up. However, she emphatically states she is not interested in quitting smoking.

PMHx: COPD, frequent UTIs

PSHx: Open cholecystectomy 20 years ago, right knee surgery for arthritis last year

Meds: Albuterol MDI, AeroBid MDI, calcium   **All:** NKDA

SHx: Smokes one pack per day, married 43 years   **GYNHx:** Normal Pap smears, no STDs

OBHx: NSVD × 3

THOUGHT QUESTIONS
- What is the differential diagnosis of urinary incontinence for this patient?
- What will you focus on with the exam?
- What labs are part of the standard workup?

Urinary incontinence can be classified into four basic types:

    stress incontinence (SI)
    urge incontinence (UI)
    overflow incontinence
    functional incontinence (due to factors that have nothing to do with the lower urinary tract and
        are often reversible)

Although this patient's history is classic for SI symptoms, you first need to rule out reversible causes of urinary incontinence – a useful mnemonic is DIAPPERS (delirium, infection, atrophic vaginitis/ urethritis, pharm, psych, endocrine (calcium, DI, DM, polydipsia), restricted mobility, stool impaction). The workup should incorporate a thorough history, PE with pelvic and neurological exam, and urinalysis. On pelvic exam you should look for a cystocele, rectocele, enterocele, or uterine prolapse.

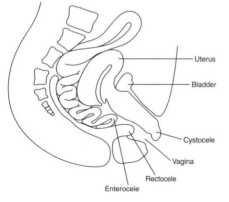

FIGURE 6-1 Pelvic floor prolapse. (Illustration by Electronic Illustrators Group.)

Uterus

Bladder

Cystocele

Vagina

Rectocele

Enterocele

Stress testing can be done with the patient standing or lying down. Ask her to cough or strain and note the amount and timing of any urine loss. A Q-tip test looks for urethral hypermobility. With the patient in the dorsal lithotomy position gently insert a sterile Q-tip lubricated with 2% lidocaine jelly into the urethra to the level of the bladder. The angle that the swab makes with the horizontal while the patient is at rest is recorded. Then ask the patient to perform a Valsalva's maneuver. If the resting and/or straining angle of the Q-tip exceeds +30 degrees, the urethrovesical junction can be considered hypermobile.

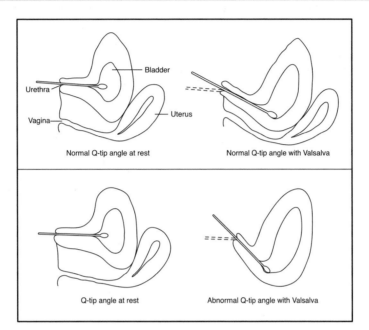

FIGURE 6-2 Q-tip test. (Illustration by Electronic Illustrators Group.)

After the exam the patient can go to the bathroom and completely empty her bladder, after which a PVR (post-void residual) should be measured.

VS: Temp 98°F BP 152/90 HR 80 Weight 192 lbs Height 5'4"

PE: *Abdomen:* soft, nontender, no masses, obese. *Speculum exam:* parous cervix, no lesions, atrophic external genitalia. *BME:* no prolapse, no cystocele or rectocele, positive urine loss with Valsalva, Q-tip test 45 degrees, no adnexal masses. *DRE:* no masses, stool guaiac negative.

Labs: *Urinalysis:* negative. *PVR:* 30cc

QUESTIONS

21. You diagnose the patient with stress incontinence based on the H&P. Which component of her history is NOT a risk factor for SI?
    A. Multiparity
    B. COPD
    C. Age
    D. Prior abdominal surgery (cholecystectomy)

22. Which treatment for SI would you begin with in this patient?
    A. Kegel exercises
    B. Urethral plug
    C. Imipramine
    D. Refer for surgery

23. Which patients should you refer to a gynecologist or urologist for further workup and treatment?
    A. Urinary tract infection
    B. No prolapse on exam
    C. Low PVR
    D. History of prior anti-incontinence surgery

24. More than 50% of incontinence patients have a mixed SI and UI. How do you decide what treatment they need?
    A. Urodynamic studies
    B. Patient tells you which type of incontinence predominates
    C. Doesn't matter as the treatment is the same anyway
    D. Trial and error

CASE 7 / MENOPAUSE

ID/CC: HT is a 56-year-old woman coming in for her annual physical.

HPI: The patient is a Vietnamese G3P3 who went through menopause three years ago. She is inquiring about hormone replacement therapy (HRT). She gets mild headaches several times a month, and rarely feels hot flashes anymore although they were severe two to three years ago. She complains of occasional vaginal itching, which can be terrible at times. She also gets frequent yeast infections and mild dyspareunia as well as decreased libido and fatigue. She has urinary incontinence episodes three to five times a week which are usually associated with coughing or running. She denies dysuria, urgency, or frequency. She feels her memory is not as good recently, and she becomes depressed or overwhelmed more easily these days.

PMHx: Hypertension, hyperlipidemia   **PSHx:** C/S × 3   **OBHx:** C/S × 3

GYNHx: Menarche age 12, menopause age 53, normal Pap smears, no STDs

Urge incontinence which is somewhat improved with meds

ROS: Intermittent mild dyspareunia

Meds: Simvastatin 20 mg per day, metoprolol 100 mg per day, calcium 500 mg per day, oxybutynin 5 mg three times a day

All: NKDA

FHx: Mother has DM, aunt had femur fracture age 66, another aunt had a radial fracture age 62, father HTN and MI age 54. No FHx CA

THOUGHT QUESTIONS
- What will you tell the patient about the pros and cons of HRT?
- What are the different kinds of HRT she can choose from?

Pros: Although all the research is not yet complete, it is generally accepted that HRT decreases HgbA1c; improves GU atrophy, incontinence, and possibly dyspareunia; treats vasomotor symptoms of menopause; and increases BMD (bone mineral density). There is also increasing evidence that indicates that HRT may protect against Alzheimer's disease and macular degeneration, and improves lipids and skin tone; it may also stabilize mood and help with memory and concentration. As of now, it is unclear whether HRT also confers cardioprotective effects apart from its effect on lipids.

Cons: Menstrual bleeding (unless on continuous), possible small increased risk of breast cancer, occasional bloating and breast tenderness, another pill to take each day, patients with a uterus must take a progesterone as well as an estrogen to protect against endometrial cancer

Available as: 1. Oral: estrogen +/– progesterone (if no uterus no need for progesterone) cyclic (10–20 days of the month) vs. continuous
2. Transdermal: patch (same effects as oral except no increase in HDL)
3. Topical (for local sxs): progesterone gel, estrogen cream

VS: Temp 97°F BP 152/79 HR 70

PE: *Lungs:* CTA, CV RRR without murmur. *Abdomen:* soft, nontender, nondistended, no HSM. *Skin:* clear. *BME:* external genitalia WNL, moderate atrophy of vaginal tissue, cervix small without lesions, uterus small and midline, no leaking urine with Valsalva. *DRE:* normal sphincter tone, guaiac negative, no masses.

> ## THOUGHT QUESTION
> • The patient is curious about all the changes she has experienced as "the menopause."

You explain that menopause results from the loss of ovarian function, which leads to decreasing cyclic estrogen levels. In medicine menopause can be defined as amenorrhea for one year + symptoms of hypoestrogenism + FSH > 40 IU/L.

The symptoms patients experience are as a result of the estrogen deficiency, and include hot flashes, headache, sleep disturbances, vaginal atrophy with dryness, dyspareunia and recurrent infections, dysuria, urgency, recurrent UTIs, difficulty concentrating, loss of short-term memory, depression, loss of libido, fatigue, and irritability. Estrogen deficiency also accelerates atherosclerosis (probably secondary to increased LDL and TC and decreased HDL), skin thinning, and osteoporosis.

> ## THOUGHT QUESTION
> • The patient is concerned about getting cancer or other bad side effects from HRT. How do you respond?

Answer:

You state that multiple studies have evaluated the potential health risks of HRT, and so far have shown:

1) slight increased risk for breast cancer
2) estrogen alone in women with a uterus confers a four to seven times increased risk for endometrial cancer; however, the simultaneous use of progestins prevents this in most cases
3) no evidence of increased gallbladder disease risk in recent case-control studies
4) no increased risk for thrombophlebitis
5) no increase in blood pressure

QUESTIONS

25. Before the patient decides whether to start HRT you review the following contraindications to HRT with the patient:
    A. Past history of thromboembolic disease
    B. Family history of endometrial cancer
    C. Hypertension
    D. Active liver disease

26. She inquires about alternatives to hormones for side effects of menopause. You reply:
    A. There are none
    B. Alternative remedies exist but are no different than placebo
    C. Alternative remedies exist but don't work as well as HRT
    D. Alternative remedies exist which are as good as or even superior to HRT

27. The patient decides to start HRT to decrease her risk for osteoporosis and treat her GU atrophy. She would like to know how likely she is to have a fracture in the future if she doesn't start HRT.
    A. No way to tell without testing her BMD
    B. Very possible
    C. Unlikely, as osteoporosis is uncommon
    D. Unlikely as she has never had a fracture herself

28. The patient happily leaves your office with a prescription for oral HRT, however calls nine months later complaining of new vaginal spotting. You tell her
    A. To make an appointment for an endometrial biopsy and ultrasound
    B. To double up her pills for a month
    C. That it is from the HRT and will resolve spontaneously
    D. To stop taking the pills immediately and that you will refer her to a gynecologic surgeon for endometrial cancer

CASE 8 / ABNORMAL PAP

ID/CC: CN is a 29-year-old patient who returns for the results of her latest Pap smear.

HPI: The patient is a G2P2 who has been followed for abnormal Pap smears. Her Pap smear history is as follows:

> four years ago: no cellular abnormality
> last year: ASCUS (abnormal squamous cells of uncertain significance), favor reactive
> six months ago: no cellular abnormality, reactive changes
> two weeks ago: LGSIL (low-grade squamous intraepithelial lesion)

The patient is surprised to hear about the LGSIL result and denies any intermenstrual or postcoital spotting. She denies pelvic pain or dyspareunia. Her aunt had endometrial cancer and she worries that this abnormal Pap puts her at risk for cancer of the uterus or ovaries. She has never had abnormal Paps before last year and has never had any treatment of her cervix. Her two deliveries were both vaginal deliveries.

PMHx: Rheumatoid arthritis, mild   **PSHx:** None

GYNHx: Paps as above, genital HSV diagnosed at age 19 with no recent outbreaks, eight lifetime partners

Meds: Motrin as needed, Acyclovir as needed   **All:** NKDA

PE: *Pelvic exam:* four 1–2 mm warty lesions on the posterior perineum (condyloma), otherwise exam WNL

THOUGHT QUESTION

- What will you advise next for the patient?

The transition time from a normal cervix to cancer can be as short as 12 months or as long as 20 years. Recommendations are for Pap smears annually once the woman is sexually active or has reached 18 years of age; these can be spaced out a bit to once every two to three years once a woman has three normal Paps in a row.

Pap smears are performed to detect preinvasive disease of the cervix. In the Bethesda cytologic reporting system potentially premalignant squamous lesions fall into three categories: ASCUS (atypical squamous cells of uncertain significance), LGSIL (low-grade squamous intraepithelial lesion), and HGSIL (high-grade squamous intraepithelial lesion). More than 5% of all Pap smears are read as ASCUS. Pap smears are screening tools, and any consistently abnormal results need to be verified with actual tissue diagnosis by taking a biopsy of the cervix during colposcopy: CIN (cervical intraepithelial neoplasia) I, II, III and CIS (carcinoma-in-situ).

20% of LGSIL Paps will have CIN II or III on colposcopic biopsies. However, up to 50% of those will regress to normal in the following year.

TABLE 8. Types of CIN

CIN	% REGRESS	% PERSIST	% PROGRESS	% INVASIVE CANCER
I	60	30	10	1
II	40	35	22	5
III	30	55	—	12

ASCUS, favor reactive: repeat Pap every 6mo: *3 WNL → routine annual Paps
                                                  *ASCUS or worse → colpo

ASCUS, favor dysplasia: colpo
ASCUS in patient with prior SIL: colpo
LGSIL: colpo
HGSIL: colpo

FIGURE 8 Algorithm for abnormal Pap smears.

You perform colposcopy on your patient, and see acetowhite epithelium consistent with CIN I. You do two biopsies and an endocervical curettage (ECC). The biopsies come back as "CIN I with HPV effect," and the ECC is negative.

THOUGHT QUESTION

• The patient returns a week later to discuss the results of her colposcopy, and wants to know whether her external warts should be treated also. "If the virus can cause cancer on my cervix, what about outside my vagina?"

Precancerous lesions of the vulva are termed vulvar intraepithelial neoplasms (VIN) and those of the vagina are termed vaginal intraepithelial neoplasms (VAIN). The lesions on the patient's perineum looked like classic genital warts (condyloma).

HPV is implicated in more than 80% of vulvar condyloma acuminata cases, and also in VIN. However, more than 85% of VIN is associated with high-risk HPV subtypes, such as 16 and 31. There are probably other inciting factors that cause VIN, such as cigarette smoking, concurrent STDs, and vulvar hygiene. In fact, only 60% of invasive vulvar cancer has detectable HPV on pathology. The most common symptom of VIN is pruritus. The lesions are usually red or brown and are often found on the intralabial grooves, posterior fourchette, and perineum. The diagnosis is made by biopsy, and VIN is treated with surgical excision, laser vaporization, or the topical chemotherapeutic agent 5-FU.

VAIN is associated with HPV 16 in more than 70% of cases. Lesions are most common in the upper one-third of the vagina, and appear as hyperkeratotic or punctate lesions on colposcopy.

The patient has a history of both HSV and external HPV. HSV outbreaks occur sporadically and last for one to three weeks. The lesions resemble blisters that then crust over and are usually quite painful. HPV lesions are present for month to years, and are described as skin-colored papules which are asymptomatic; the papules can be as small as skin tags, or can be exophytic, congruent, and quite extensive.

QUESTIONS

29. What treatment option would be best for this patient?
    A. Cone biopsy in the OR
    B. Cryotherapy
    C. LEEP
    D. Herbal treatments to the cervix

30. Would your management be any different if she were on high doses of prednisone for her rheumatoid arthritis?
    A. Less risk of progression of cervical disease so next Pap due in one year
    B. More risk for progression of cervical changes and need to treat more aggressively
    C. No effect on cervical cell abnormalities
    D. RA is protective against cervical cancer

31. She asks what the "HPV effect" means. You reply that:
    A. HPV is detected in most women with cervical neoplasia
    B. "HPV effect" is because of her history of genital herpes
    C. Since she doesn't have large external genital warts it must be an error
    D. HPV on the biopsy is ominous and means she needs especially aggressive treatment to avoid invasive cervical cancer

32. After treatment of the cervix, when should she have her next Pap smear?
    A. Next week
    B. Three months
    C. One year
    D. Pap smears aren't a good screening tool after cervical treatment/surgery

ID/CC: DP is a 17-year-old female patient who comes in for a school physical. During routine questioning she reports being sexually active for one year.

HPI: The patient admits that she only occasionally uses contraception, because "it seems like too much of a hassle and I don't know what the different kinds are." When you offer to review the birth control management (BCM) options available, she is very interested. She denies any dyspareunia or vaginal discharge.

PMHx: None   **PSHx:** Knee surgery age 15

GYNHx: No prior Pap smears, regular heavy periods with severe cramping, three lifetime partners

OBHx: Nullipara   **Meds:** Motrin as needed   **All:** NKDA   **FHx:** HTN

SHx: One pack of cigarettes per week, occasional marijuana

THOUGHT QUESTIONS

• What are the main classes of BCM?

• How will you counsel her in terms of risk factors and choice of BCM?

Contraceptive methods can be divided up into six main classes:

1) hormonal: progesterone only, progesterone-estrogen pills, shots (Norplant – not currently available)
2) IUD
3) barrier methods: diaphragm, cervical cap, condoms
4) withdrawal
5) natural family planning
6) permanent sterilization: vasectomy, tubal ligation

In this nulliparous teenager, sterilization and natural family planning are probably not indicated. Her risk for contracting STDs is high enough that an IUD would be unadvisable at this point. Therefore, helping the patient choose between the different hormonal methods and barrier methods should be the focus of this visit.

Hormonal methods are somewhat more efficacious than barrier methods (95% to 99% vs. 80% to 85% effective) and ideally the patient will be able to combine condoms with another method for improved protection against STDs. The progesterone injectable (Depo-Provera) is easy and confidential, and will likely decrease her menstrual flow after one or two shots, however many patients find the menstrual irregularities and other minor side effects such as headaches, three- to four-pound weight gain, and possible mood changes inconvenient. Birth control pills are great at making periods regular and light, but require the patient to remember to take a pill every day and some teenagers do not want their parents to find the pills.

TABLE 9. Birth Control Methods							
	PILLS	CONDOM	DMPA	DIAPHRAGM	IUD	BTL	VASECTOMY
Efficacy	95%	86%	99%	80%	99%	99.5%	99.9%
Dosing Frequency	daily	each time	3 months	each time	10 years	once	once
Confidentiality	moderate	moderate	high	moderate	high	high	high
Rapid return to fertility	yes	yes	no	yes	yes	no	no
Regular cycle	yes	yes	no	yes	yes	yes	yes
Advantages	high efficacy	available STD protect	high efficacy convenient	no hormone	high efficacy	high efficacy	high efficacy no work
Disadvantages	daily	use each time cost	bleeding	fitting	initial cost	cost	cost bleeding

(DMPA = Depo Provera, IUD = intrauterine device, BTL = bilateral tubal ligation)

VS: Temp 98°F BP 130/82 HR 95

PE: Lungs CTA, CV RRR without murmur, abdomen benign. *Speculum exam:* small os with yellow-white discharge, no lesions. *BME:* small anteverted uterus, no adnexal masses or tenderness

Labs: Hct 33.3, U/A negative, βhCG negative, chlamydia positive, Pap WNL

THOUGHT QUESTION
• As the patient has no symptoms or discharge, does she need treatment for the positive chlamydia swab?

Chlamydia is endemic in the United States now, and can be associated with a number of serious complications in women, including PID, a tubo-ovarian abscess, and infertility. Chlamydia is a reportable disease and can be spread to other partners quite easily. The treatments of choice include doxycycline 100 mg twice a day for seven days, or azithromycin 1 gm orally once, or ofloxacin 300 mg twice a day for seven days. The patient and her partner should also be treated for possible gonorrhea, as the two infections commonly coexist. Gonorrhea can be treated with ceftriaxone, ofloxacin, or ciprofloxacin, all in a one-time dose.

QUESTIONS

33. Your patient decides she would like OCPs (oral contraceptive pills) as her friends say their acne improves with OCPs. What other noncontraceptive benefits do OCPs confer?
    A. Decreased risk of stomach cancer
    B. Decreased incidence of PID (pelvic inflammatory disease)
    C. Improved energy
    D. Fewer varicose veins

34. After the patient has spoken with you for some time you recheck her BP and it is 110/70. To effectively counsel her about the risks or contraindications for OCPs you review:
    A. Family history MI
    B. History of DVT/PE
    C. Personal history of tobacco use
    D. Personal history of street drug use

35. The patient leaves your office with a prescription for OCPs, however four months later is back in your office. She never filled the prescription and had unprotected intercourse the previous night. She wants the "day-after pill." You review the requirements for emergency contraception with the patient:
    A. Unprotected intercourse within 24 hours
    B. Positive pregnancy test
    C. No prior history of DVT
    D. Normal liver function

36. This time the patient asks for a Depo-Provera shot at the end of the visit. Side effects include all of the following except:
    A. Irregular bleeding
    B. Headache
    C. Dizziness
    D. Hirsutism

CASE 10 / STDs

ID/CC: PD is a 27-year-old female patient who comes into the clinic with her boyfriend. She is complaining of yellow vaginal discharge.

HPI: The patient has had dysuria, pelvic pain, and yellow discharge for a week. She denies any nausea or vomiting but has had subjective fevers. Her boyfriend is without complaints. They have been together for 18 months and are planning on trying to have a child soon. Her LMP was 10 days ago. She has a history of genital herpes but has not had an outbreak for five months. She uses OCPs and does not use condoms.

PMHx: None   **PSHx:** None   **Meds:** None   **All:** NKDA   **OBHx:** Nullipara

GYNHx: Trichomoniasis age 18, HSV since age 21 with one to two outbreaks a year, normal Paps

---

> ### THOUGHT QUESTIONS
> - What are the most common STDs?
> - How do you diagnose and treat them?

One in four Americans experience an STD during their lifetime.

TABLE 10. Common STDs

STD	INCIDENCE*	DIAGNOSIS	TREATMENT
Gonorrhea (Neisseria gonorrhea)	650,000	culture, ELISA DFA, DNA probe	ceftriaxone 125 mg intramuscular cefixime 400 mg by mouth ciprofloxacin 500 mg by mouth
Chlamydia (Chlamydia trachomatis)	3 million	culture, ELISA DFA, DNA probe	doxycycline 100 mg twice a day for seven days azithromycin 1 gm by mouth erythromycin, ofloxacin
Herpes (Herpes simplex virus)	1 million	Tzanck smear culture PE	acyclovir 400 mg by mouth three times a day famciclovir 250 mg by mouth three times a day valacyclovir 1 gm by mouth twice a day
Syphilis (Treponema pallidum)	70,000	VDRL, RPR Dark field microscopy MHA-TP, FTA-ABS	penicillin as per stage
Trichomoniasis (Trichomonas vaginalis)	5 million	wet mount, culture	metronidazole 2 gm by mouth
HPV (extern) (Human papilloma virus)	5.5 million	PE, Pap smear	podophyllin, imiquimod, TCA, cryotherapy, surgery

(*Incidence = # new cases/year in U.S.)

VS: Temp 100.6°F BP 106/68 HR 110 RR 14

PE: Lungs CTA, CV sinus tachycardia without murmur. Abdomen soft, mild tenderness to palpation BLQ, no CVAT. *SSE:* friable cervix with yellow discharge from os, no lesions seen. *BME:* EG WNL, + CMT, uterus anteverted and normal size, mild bilateral adnexal tenderness without masses

THOUGHT QUESTION
- Which STDs, if any, are reportable?

In the United States, each state has a different list of reportable diseases, but all use the uniform CDC criteria for reporting cases. The CDC requires state health departments to report all cases of: AIDS, chlamydia, chancroid, gonorrhea, syphilis, hepatitis B, hepatitis C. STDs that are not reportable include herpes, HPV, lymphogranuloma venereum, granuloma inguinale, nongonococcal urethritis, and PID.

Data for nationally reportable diseases are published weekly in the *Morbidity and Mortality Weekly Report*. Health officials rely on doctors and clinics to report the occurrence of infectious diseases so that incidence and prevalence trends can be accurately monitored and the effectiveness of treatments can be evaluated, including antibiotic resistance and particularly high-risk populations.

THOUGHT QUESTION
- The patient would like a prescription for "those new herpes medicines" to treat her genital herpes once and for all. What medicine does she mean?

There is no medication that exists so far to eradicate latent herpes virus. Antiviral medications such as acyclovir reduce the severity and duration of symptoms, and also appear to reduce the number of outbreaks if taken prophylactically. Antiviral medication does not affect the risk, frequency, or severity of recurrences after the drug is discontinued.

Transmission of HSV occurs via direct contact with infected secretions. After resolution of the primary episode the virus remains latent in the dorsal nerve root ganglia and can be reactivated by stress, trauma, menstruation, intercourse, and sunlight, among others. Before lesions appear, paresthesias and burning may occur. Vesicles then appear, enlarge, and rupture to form shallow, painful ulcerations, which eventually crust over and heal.

QUESTIONS

37. You send a culture of the discharge, and a Gram's stain shows gram-negative diplococci. The wet mount and KOH prep are negative. The most common complication of gonorrhea in women is:
    A. Bartholin's abscess
    B. Perihepatitis (Fitz-Hugh-Curtis syndrome)
    C. Conjunctivitis
    D. PID

38. Given the patient's complete H&P you diagnose her with:
    A. PID
    B. Gonococcal cervicitis
    C. Chlamydial cervicitis
    D. Bacterial vaginosis

39. Criteria for hospitalization for treatment of her diagnosis include:
    A. Unable to follow or tolerate outpatient oral regimen
    B. Adnexal tenderness
    C. History of PID in past
    D. History of infertility

40. The patient wants to know if her chances of becoming pregnant will be affected. You tell her that
    A. Her risk for ectopic pregnancy is doubled
    B. 50% of women are infertile after three episodes
    C. Because her symptoms are worsening, her risk for infertility is higher
    D. Her fertility is not affected as long as she doesn't develop a TOA (tubo-ovarian abscess)

ID/CC: One of your patients, a 13-month-old, is added to your drop-in slot because of his "barky cough."

HPI: JS is a previously healthy baby that you have been seeing in your continuity practice since birth (you first met him in the delivery room!). Last evening he had a temperature of 100.4°F axillary and was a little cranky with a runny nose and watery eyes. The parents were awakened at 3 a.m. by his cough that sounded like barking and an unusually course cry. Since then JS has been fussy, has been nursing a little but not eating his usual foods, and continues with his hoarse voice and coughing. His parents are worried that he is having trouble breathing, but he seemed to calm down a bit in the car.

PMHx: No antibiotic use; no history of noisy breathing.   **Meds:** Tylenol four hours prior

All: NKDA   **Birth Hx:** Full-term, NSVD, went home with mom two days postpartum.

DevHx: Sat alone at 7 months, walked on own one week ago. Says dada/mama.

Immunizations: UTD including 12-month vaccinations.

DietHx: Breastfed only through 6 months; now eats variety of table foods plus cow's milk (since 12 months) and comfort nursing. No history of feeding abnormalities.

FHx: dad with asthma

THOUGHT QUESTION
- What portions of the physical exam are most important for this patient?

For any urgent respiratory symptom in a young child, it is most crucial to establish the presence or absence of "respiratory distress." Because young children have a very small caliber upper airway, they are more vulnerable to airway occlusion and will show increased work of breathing if compromised. Tachypnea is the first sign of increased respiratory demand. (The normal respiratory rate for a 1- to 4-year-old is 20–30.) Accessory muscle use may also be evident. Retractions can be seen in the intercostal, subcostal, supra-sternal, and supraclavicular regions. Nasal flaring will be seen in a more distressed child. Grunting, the child's attempt to create positive end-expiratory pressure, is an ominous sign. The child's position can also give clues: open mouth breathing while sitting forward opens the supra-glottic airway. Cyanosis, ineffective respiratory effort, and altered level of consciousness signify impending respiratory failure and warrant intubation.

CASE CONTINUED

The mom carries JS into the room; he is vigorous and has a full, stridorous cry with intermittent barky coughs.

VS: Temp 38.8°C rectal HR 140 RR 34 O_2 Saturation 97% on RA

PE: *HEENT:* crying tears, clear rhinorrhea, TMs erythematous but mobile with no effusion, oropharynx not visualized. Anterior fontanel fingertip, flat. *Neck:* no LAD CV: rate at 140, regular, no M/R/G. *Resp:* Initially, stridorous crying. Once quiet in mom's lap, no stridor at rest; intermittent coughing. Mild suprasternal retractions only. Lungs are clear to auscultation without wheeze, good air movement. *Abdomen:* Soft, NABS. *Extremities:* warm/well-perfused. *Neuro:* Cranky but consolable; age appropriate. You observe the baby nursing without difficulty. *Skin:* no rash, normal turgor.

The most common causes of acute upper airway obstruction in the 6-month-old to 3-year-old are croup, epiglottitis, and foreign-body aspiration. Epiglottitis (supraglottitis) has become less common with the use of the Hib vaccine. It is characterized by sore throat, high fever, toxic appearance, and progressive difficulty swallowing (possibly with extensive drooling). Epiglottitis can also be caused by *Strep. pneumoniae* and *Staph. aureus*; in all cases blood cultures are positive 80–90% of the time. If epiglottitis is suspected, no agitating procedures (such as rectal exam, separation from parent, or forcible examination of the oropharynx) should be done.

Foreign-body aspiration should always be a consideration in the evaluation of a young child with stridor. More than 50% of the time, there is no history of choking or foreign body ingestion. Symptoms are usually sudden in onset in an afebrile child. Radiographs with lateral decubitus films are essential in making this diagnosis.

Croup (viral laryngotracheobronchitis) accounts for 90% of cases with stridor and fever. It is a diffuse swelling of the subglottic region; parainfluenza is most commonly responsible. It is associated with moderate fever and URI symptoms. Symptoms usually worsen for three days, then improve.

This patient has a classic presentation of croup and needs no further diagnostic studies.

QUESTIONS

41. Which of the following is recommended treatment for this patient?
    A. Racemic epinephrine 0.25% solution via nebulizer followed by observation for two hours
    B. Education, recommendation for cool-mist therapy, follow-up in 24 hours by phone or visit
    C. Dexamethasone 0.6 mg/kg IM, followed by observation for four hours
    D. Humidified oxygen, and lateral neck radiographs when the baby is calm

42. What radiograph finding would be most common in our patient?
    A. The steeple sign
    B. Flattened diaphragms
    C. Deviated trachea
    D. Fluffy bilateral infiltrates

43. Bacterial tracheitis differs from croup in that:
    A. It affects a different age range
    B. It is an infection of a different part of the airway
    C. It does not cause stridor
    D. The children usually have a very toxic appearance and a high fever

44. All of the following are true regarding upper airway diseases except:
    A. Retropharyngeal abscesses occur most commonly in children under 3.
    B. Peritonsillar abscesses often cause trismus (pain with opening the mouth) and "hot-potato" phonation.
    C. 65% of deaths due to foreign-body aspiration are in infants under 12 months
    D. Chronic stridor in a young infant is most commonly foreign-body aspiration

CASE 12 / NEWBORN ISSUES

ID/CC: A healthy 22-year-old single woman gives birth to a boy by NSVD, her first baby. You are seeing her the following day for a postpartum check and she has a lot of questions!

HPI: NM recently moved from another city and received most of her prenatal care elsewhere, although she brought her lab results with her. Her pregnancy was unplanned; the father is currently not involved. Her labor and delivery were uncomplicated, and she is planning on going home the following day. She asks, "What do you think about circumcision?" and "What's the deal with breastfeeding?"

Prenatal Hx: All PNL within normal limits; GC/chlamydia negative   **Meds:** Prenatal vitamins, iron

All: NKDA   **Habits:** No tobacco, alcohol, or recreational drugs

SHx: NM lives in a two-bedroom apartment that she is sharing with her aunt. She plans to stay with the baby for at least three months, and then try to find a part-time job. She is getting some financial support from her father. She has not been sexually active since moving to the area.

THOUGHT QUESTION
- How do you discuss the topic of circumcision with expectant and new parents?

First, it is ideal to have a series of conversations with any involved parents. It is best to first hear the parents' ideas about circumcision: What have they been told? Are their family members circumcised? Do they have a preference already? Next, it's appropriate to introduce a little of the history of circumcision. Circumcision has been present since 3000 BC and has been accepted intermittently by cultures since then. Historical justifications for circumcision have been: 1) it promotes health, 2) it is aesthetically pleasing, 3) it is the custom. In the United States, circumcision was the custom from the late 1800s through the 1980s, at which point 80% of newborn boys were circumcised. Since then, the practice has fallen off; recently about 45% of boys in North America are circumcised (60–65% of boys in the United States).

Health issues: Circumcision has been touted as a way to prevent balanitis, phimosis, and dyspareunia, and decrease incidence of urinary tract infection and pyelonephritis. Retrospective analysis does suggest a higher incidence of pyelonephritis and UTI in the uncircumcised infant until 9 months of age. Circumcision may decrease the already low risk of cancer of the penis. Cervical cancer may be more common in partners of uncircumcised males, but likely not in those who practice good hygiene. Sexually transmitted diseases are more common in uncircumcised males, although the effects of hygiene are not known. With normal bathing, an intact foreskin is easy to care for. Although circumcision is still being studied, there is no definitive literature to indicate a clear medical recommendation to circumcise every male infant. Circumcision is much less common in most other developed countries.

The procedure: It is important to discuss the logistics of circumcision, including who will perform it, how long it will take, and what care is expected afterwards. Institutions and physicians vary as to circumcision practices. In many institutions, obstetricians or pediatricians perform them prior to baby's discharge from the hospital. The outpatient family practice doctor may circumcise at the first weight check; religious circumcisions are often later. Although circumcision techniques vary, the procedure shouldn't take longer than 10 minutes. Care afterward includes ointment and gauze to the exposed glans to prevent the diaper from sticking; normal granulation tissue should appear within two days.

CASE CONTINUED

The mother explains that the father was circumcised, but that she doesn't want the baby to have a surgery that isn't necessary. She explains that the baby breastfed immediately after birth for about 10 minutes, but he hasn't wanted to nurse much since then. She then says, "I think that breastfeeding is going to be harder than I thought. Is it really better than formula?"

THOUGHT QUESTION
• In what ways is breastfeeding different from formula feeding?

Breast milk provides the best nutrition for the baby; formula is an inferior substitution. The benefits of breastfeeding to the baby are numerous and include: reduced food allergy, reduced otitis media, reduced gastroenteritis and respiratory infections, less constipation, and possible enhanced neurodevelopment. Breast milk is less costly and more convenient than formula. The mother-infant pair will show increased bonding and more responsive child-rearing behaviors. In the mother, breastfeeding stimulates the release of oxytocin, which helps contract the uterus to prepregnancy size. It also confers a lower risk of breast cancer for the mother.

CASE CONTINUED

The mother asks you to watch her breastfeed, and you observe the baby latch on to the nipple. You explain that proper latching is the most important element for successful breastfeeding and assist with a proper latch. You see the baby's ears wiggle with suckling and know the positioning is correct!

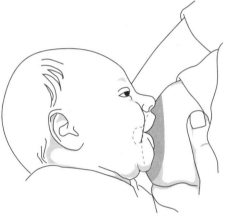

FIGURE 12 Proper positioning of the baby on the breast. (Illustration by Shawn Girsberger Graphic Design.)

lips everted, areola site of latch-on, base of nipple entirely in baby's mouth

QUESTIONS

45. In the uncircumcised male, when will the foreskin be naturally fully retractable?
    A. In 50% of boys by age 12 months
    B. In 90% of boys by age 2 years
    C. In 90% of boys by age 3 years
    D. In 95% of boys by age 5 years

46. Regarding analgesia for neonatal circumcision, which of the following is correct?
    A. Pain experienced by infants during circumcision is inconsequential; a sugar-water nipple is the best pacifier
    B. Lidocaine-prilocaine cream, applied to the penis and foreskin for 60 to 80 minutes prior to circumcision, is the most effective way to diminish the pain response
    C. Dorsal penile nerve block is not recommended due to the risk of penile necrosis
    D. Untreated pain from circumcision has been linked to short-term alterations in sleeping, feeding, and crying in the infant

47. Which of the following is not a component of breast milk?
    A. A higher proportion of casein than whey
    B. B- and T-lymphocytes, macrophages, and neutrophils
    C. Cholesterol in a higher proportion than cow's milk or formula
    D. Secretory IgA, lipase, and a satiety factor

48. Which of the following is not a contraindication of breastfeeding?
    A. Active, untreated tuberculosis infection in the mother
    B. Active chicken pox infection in the mother
    C. Infant of less than 34 weeks gestation
    D. Mother who is HIV+

CASE 13 / "MY SON HAS TROUBLE AT SCHOOL"

ID/CC: A 35-year-old woman comes in for her Pap/pelvic exam and says, "My son is really having trouble at school."

HPI: Your patient describes what's been going on. Since her 7-year-old, SA, started first grade, he has been getting into trouble in his classroom. He squirms a lot and has not been focusing well on writing or quiet work. His teachers say that he is easily distractible and gets up a lot when he is supposed to stay seated.

THOUGHT QUESTION

• What should you do now?

In a child who is having academic or social difficulties at school, it is worthwhile to first schedule an appointment with the parent(s), then schedule a separate visit to include the child.

The parents can then give a thorough history along with their perspective, then you can observe and interview the child, depending on the age.

CASE CONTINUED

You schedule an appointment in two weeks with SA's mother and father for a detailed history. They report that he has always been "active," running around, and is sensitive to his environment. His kindergarten teachers noted that he "had a lot of energy" and was physical with his friends. This year, he has seemed less happy to go to school. When he is at home, he listens to his parents pretty well, although he has to be reminded sometimes. Their discipline method is revocation of privileges. He has a younger sister who is "much calmer"; they get along. His parents feel that he is a sweet but excitable boy who needs a quieter environment at school. He had a normal vision and hearing test within the previous six months.

You meet with SA the next week; he agrees that it is hard for him to sit still in class, and that they don't have enough time for recess. He says he doesn't like to write. He cooperates with your exam and is willing to chat and answer questions. His parents come back in and ask you, "So, does he have ADD?"

THOUGHT QUESTION

• How do you diagnose ADD (now known as ADHD)?

Any child having difficulty at school should first be screened for hearing, vision, and speech deficits. "Learning disabilities" like dyslexia, visual processing problems, and other disorders such as sensory integration dysfunction may also be coexistent with or manifest as symptoms of ADHD. It may be difficult to separate these issues; psychological testing may be needed to clarify the etiology of the symptoms. Attention deficit hyperactivity disorder is a common syndrome that may affect up to 10% of school age children. It is characterized by hyperactivity, impulsivity, and inattention that are beyond normal for the child's developmental level. The DSM-IV diagnostic criteria are used as a diagnostic tool for establishing the presence of ADHD. These abbreviated criteria are shown in Table 13. It is helpful to have the parent and teacher fill out a questionnaire regarding these behaviors. However, the diagnosis is clearly an inexact science. Symptoms of inattention and hyperactivity-impulsivity can only be described subjectively. What happens when the impairment from the symptoms is only at school, but the impairment is significant? These issues make it important to gather as much information as possible, hopefully including a school observation. No objective test can be used to confirm the diagnosis; it is solely a clinical diagnosis.

CASE CONTINUED

The medical student working in your office is able to do a school observation with the parents' consent, and report back to you. The class had 24 students, arranged in pod-like groups. The son did get up often during activities that he disliked, such as writing. He made several careless mistakes, was distracted by

TABLE 13. Abbreviated Diagnostic Criteria for ADHD (DSM-IV) (Need A, B, C, D, and E)

A. Either (1) or (2):
   (1) Six (or more) symptoms of inattention that have persisted for at least six months to a degree that is maladaptive and inconsistent with developmental level (see DSM-IV for checklist).
   (2) Six (or more) symptoms of hyperactivity-impulsivity that have persisted for at least six months to a degree that is maladaptive and inconsistent with developmental level (see DSM-IV for checklist).
B. Hyperactive-impulsive or inattentive symptoms that caused impairment or were present before age 7 years.
C. Impairment from the symptoms is present in two or more settings (e.g., at school [or work] and at home).
D. There must be clear evidence of clinically significant impairment in social, academic, or occupational functioning.
E. The symptoms do not occur exclusively during the course of pervasive developmental disorder, schizophrenia, or other psychotic disorder and are not better accounted for by another mental disorder (e.g., mood disorder, anxiety disorder, dissociative disorder, or a personality disorder).

other kids, and fidgeted quite often. He was able to concentrate quietly and at length during other activities like math and blocks. She did not notice any other criteria behaviors. Based on her assessment, your assessment of the child in the office, the teacher's report, and the parental report, you decide that he doesn't meet criteria for ADHD now. He does have several behaviors and school habits that are counterproductive. You counsel the parents on techniques to assist his study habits and write a letter to the school with similar recommendations. He will begin working with the educational consultant at school to assist with his writing. You make a follow-up appointment for three months hence to re-evaluate the situation.

THOUGHT QUESTION
- In a child who does meet criteria for ADHD, what are the treatment options?

Stimulants are the main pharmacologic therapy for ADHD. These include methylphenidate (Ritalin), dextroamphetamine, and pemoline—all of these have been shown to reduce core symptoms of ADHD. Bupropion (an atypical antidepressant) is showing promise as an alternative therapy. Clonidine and TCAs have limited evidence but may be effective. Behavioral therapy treatment has to date not been shown to reduce symptoms, unless combined with methylphenidate. Other treatments such as cognitive treatment, restrictive or supplemental diets, amino acid supplementation, allergy treatments, and megavitamins have not been shown to be effective in controlled studies.

CASE CONTINUED

Your patient and family return in three months. The parents have not noticed a change at home, but the teachers feel that some progress is being made. The school is using a quiet study booth for all individual work, and has noticed an improvement in ability to focus. Your patient's school work has shown significant improvement. You all agree to reassess with a repeat observation in another three months unless something else comes up.

QUESTIONS

49. Adverse effects of methylphenidate, dextroamphetamine, and pemoline include all of the following except:
    A. Increased appetite
    B. Insomnia
    C. Abdominal pain
    D. Tachycardia

50. ADHD affects:
    A. Boys and girls equally
    B. Boys more than girls
    C. Girls more than boys
    D. Boys and girls equally until age 10, then predominantly boys.

51. Common comorbidities in children with ADHD include all of the following except:
    A. Oppositional-defiant disorder
    B. Alcohol abuse
    C. Nocturnal enuresis
    D. Conduct disorder
    E. Learning disabilities (such as dyslexia)

52. Children diagnosed with ADHD:
    A. Usually have total regression of their symptoms by adolescence
    B. Usually have total regression of their symptoms by adulthood
    C. May carry the diagnosis to adulthood
    D. Should be placed in special-education classrooms

CASE 14 / AMENORRHEA IN AN ADOLESCENT

ID/CC: WP is a 12-year-old female brought in for her school physical exam by her mother

HPI: WP is a 12-year-old Latina entering the sixth grade. She is accompanied by her mother and 24-month-old half-brother. WP is fluent in English, although it is her second language, and her mother speaks enough English to complete the medical history. She has no complaints or concerns of her own, but her mother is concerned that WP has not had her period for two months, especially since the patient's aunts, cousins, and mother had early onset of menarche at 10 and 11 years. Menarche for this patient was five months ago, with three irregular episodes of vaginal bleeding/spotting, lasting between three to seven days, no dysmenorrhea. The mother is also worried that the patient is "picky" when she eats, and looks "too skinny." The patient does not think she is "skinny," but does think that her mother is "fat."

PMHx: None   **PSHx:** Tonsillectomy at 3 years old   **Meds:** None

All: NKDA   **FHx:** Mother with menarche at 10 years old

SHx: Entering sixth grade, lives with mother and half-brother, no contact with father, mother emigrated to the United States from El Salvador. Likes art class, enjoys playing with younger brother, has friends at school. Patient does not think she is fat, but does admit fear of becoming fat; her friends share similar views. She can name several foods that she likes.

Family Dynamics: Mother answers questions when asked to patient. Little brother running about room, turning the water faucet on and off; WP tries to catch little brother to control him. Mother tells WP to sit still, while allowing little brother to continue running around the examination room.

ROS: Unremarkable   **VS:** Temp 37°C BP 108/60 HR 80 RR 18

PE: Height 56 inches or 144 cm (10 to 25 %ile) Weight 35 kg or 77 lb. (10 to 25 %ile). *Gen:* pleasant, NAD, appropriate behavior. *CV:* RRR no murmurs, nl S1 S2. *Chest:* CTA bilaterally. *Back:* no scoliotic curves. *Extremities:* wnl. *Reflexes:* 2+ symmetric biceps and patellar.

THOUGHT QUESTIONS
- Does this patient have an eating disorder?
- How would you manage the patient at this point?

The clinical picture is suggestive of an eating disorder, specifically anorexia nervosa; WP, however, at this point in time, does not meet the diagnostic criteria for anorexia. The DSM-IV criteria are

- refusal to maintain body weight over a minimal normal weight for age and height (weight less than 85% of expected)
- intense fear of becoming fat even though underweight
- disturbed body image or denial of seriousness of low body weight
- absence of three consecutive menstrual periods (secondary amenorrhea for three months)

The patient exhibits one of these characteristics—fear of becoming fat, even though at normal weight. She does not have an exceedingly low body weight, nor does she have a disturbed body image. Her amenorrhea at this time may merely be dysfunctional uterine bleeding secondary to the adjustments of the hypothalamic-pituitary axis during puberty, especially since the patient has not yet established a regular menstrual cycle.

Even though the patient does not have a diagnosis of anorexia, she should have close follow-up to ensure that menses resume, weight is not dropping, and anorexia does not develop. Nutritional counseling should be started with this patient and her family, as well as further investigation into the eating lifestyles of this family.

CASE CONTINUED

The patient returns for follow-up in three months and in six months. Patient's mother reports that WP's last menstrual cycle occurred three months ago. The following is her growth chart:

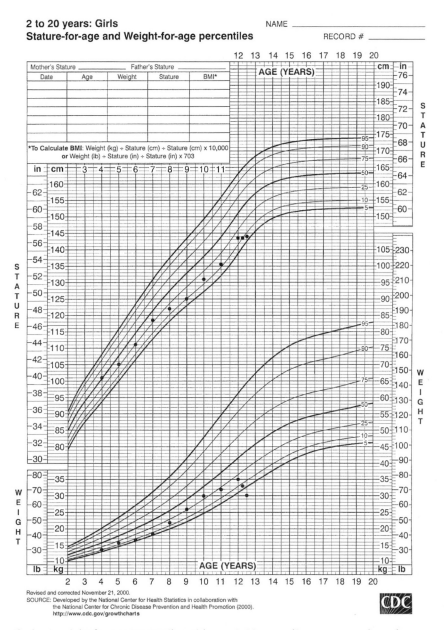

2 to 20 years: Girls
Stature-for-age and Weight-for-age percentiles

NAME _____

RECORD # _____

FIGURE 14 CDC growth chart weight-for-age percentiles, girls age 2–20 years. (Source: www.cdc.gov.)

QUESTIONS

53. A patient with anorexia nervosa may exhibit all of the following physical features EXCEPT:
    A. Temporal wasting
    B. Osteoporosis
    C. Impaired thermal regulation
    D. Vitiligo

54. List the following causes of mortality in adolescents in order of frequency:
    i.   Suicides
    ii. Childhood leukemias
    iii. Motor vehicle accidents
    iv. Homicides
    A. i, iii, iv, ii
    B. i, iv, ii, iii
    C. iii, iv, i, ii
    D. iii, i, iv, ii

55. All of the following are laboratory data that should be obtained for this patient EXCEPT:
    A. Basic metabolic panel
    B. Liver function tests
    C. Hemoglobin A1C
    D. Complete blood count

56. Which of the following questions is appropriate in obtaining a history from an adolescent patient?
    A. What kinds of activities do you like and participate in at school?
    B. Have you used or experimented with any kinds of drugs—like cigarettes, marijuana, alcohol, or any other types of drugs?
    C. Do you ever feel down or depressed?
    D. All of the above

CASE 15 / LEFT ARM PAIN IN A 3-YEAR-OLD BOY

ID/CC: NB is a 3-year-old Caucasian boy with left arm pain brought to the acute care clinic by his mother

HPI: The mother notes that NB started complaining two days ago that his arm hurt. She thinks the pain developed after the patient was playing in the park with some other children. She did not see the injury occur because she was talking to another child's mother at the park. She waited to bring him to the doctor because their family is new in town, and do not currently have a family doctor. She tells you also that the patient has always been "accident-prone"; she is never surprised when he is injured because he is "a typical boy."

PMHx: None   **Meds:** Children's acetaminophen   **All:** Cephalosporins cause a rash

ROS: Mother denies that the patient has any other symptoms   **FHx:** Noncontributory

SHx: Lives in a one-bedroom apartment with mother, father, and two half-sisters, 5-year-old and 6-year-old (same biological mother, but different biological fathers). Not enrolled in preschool, parents are trying to home school all three children. Parents unemployed, on AFDC. No other family in the area.

VS: Temp 36.8°C HR 120

PE: *Gen:* thin, disheveled boy, clinging to mother, crying, not moving left arm. *Skin:* two circular brown ecchymoses (2 cm diameter) over the patella bilaterally, and one circular yellow ecchymosis (1 cm diameter) distal to the right olecranon process. *HEENT:* WNL. *Neck:* supple, full ROM. *CV:* RRR no murmurs. *Chest:* CTA bilaterally. *Abdomen:* benign. *Back:* two linear abrasions 4 cm in length over lumbosacral area and buttocks. *Extremities:* left arm held in 90 degree flexed position close to the patient's body, with obvious guarding of that extremity; patient refuses to move or reach for objects with the left arm; no obvious deformity/swelling/discoloration; difficult to ascertain tenderness because the patient cries with any palpation of the left extremity, most tenderness seems to be located at the left elbow; left shoulder range of motion intact, as well as left wrist and digits; radial pulses 2+ bilaterally

---

THOUGHT QUESTIONS

- What workup should be done to evaluate the patient's injury?
- What is the most likely diagnosis?

A left arm radiograph should be obtained to rule out any fractures. The most likely diagnosis is radial head subluxation. This diagnosis should not be assumed, however, since the mechanism of injury was unwitnessed. Radial head subluxation ("nursemaid's elbow") is most common in toddlers, secondary to ligament laxity, and usually occurs secondary to a "pulling" mechanism (i.e., adult holding hands with a toddler and "pulling" the child along). Reduction of a radial head subluxation occurs by extending and supinating the affected forearm, while maintaining firm pressure on the radial head at the elbow. A "click" can be felt when the radial head relocates, indicating a successful reduction.

CASE CONTINUED

A left arm radiograph reveals no fractures. NB is diagnosed with a left radial head subluxation, and it is reduced. After 30 minutes, the patient stops crying and begins to move his left arm again. The patient's mother is grateful for the medical services, and is anxious to leave, saying that she must return home because her two daughters are at home alone. Because of the history and physical examination, however, they are asked to stay for further evaluation.

THOUGHT QUESTIONS
- Why are they asked to stay?
- What findings in the history and physical examination warrant an extended visit?
- What further workup is needed?

NB and his mother are asked to stay because the history and physical examination are suspicious for child abuse. Findings in the history which arouse suspicion are the delay in seeking medical care, inadequate supervision of the child when the injury occurred, and inadequate supervision of two young daughters at home alone. The injury itself is not suspicious for abuse, as nursemaid's elbow occurs frequently in toddlers. The linear abrasions on the back and buttocks, however, are suspicious for being struck with an object, such as a stick. The bruises on the hard surfaces of the extremities are age-appropriate developmental injuries (falling in a toddler), and are not suspicious for abuse. Further workup entails additional history into the injuries, physical findings, social support network, and a report to state child protective services agencies. If the child appears to be in an unsafe situation, temporary hospitalization or placement with emergency foster care can be obtained with the help of social workers. At the very minimum, further history must be obtained in this case. The law mandates that physicians must report any suspected case of child abuse.

QUESTIONS

57. Which of the following findings is not consistent with suspected child abuse?
    A. Posterior rib fractures in a 4-year-old girl
    B. Thoracic spinous process fracture in a 3-year-old boy
    C. Transverse radial fracture in a 10-year-old boy
    D. Metaphysial ("bucket-handle," "corner," or "chip") fracture of the tibia in a 6-year-old girl

58. Which of the following is not true regarding physician reporting of child abuse?
    A. The law only requires reporting of proven cases of child abuse
    B. Physicians who make an unbiased report of suspected abuse are protected from lawsuits
    C. The reportable forms of abuse are defined under state law, making child abuse a legal finding, and not a diagnosis
    D. Careful documentation of clear and specific objective findings, including photographs, must be made in the medical record whenever child abuse is suspected

59. Which form of child abuse has the greatest reported incidence?
    A. Sexual abuse
    B. Emotional abuse
    C. Physical abuse
    D. Neglect

60. Which of the following statements regarding child abuse is true?
    A. Child abuse is more likely to occur in families where spousal abuse occurs
    B. Most child abuse occurs in daycare and foster-care settings
    C. Child abuse is more likely to be perpetrated by a stranger to the child
    D. The incidence of child abuse is greater in urban settings than in rural environments

ID/CC: AH is a 3-day-old girl brought to her family doctor with yellow eyes

HPI: AH is 3 days old, delivered by uncomplicated vaginal delivery at term to a 26-year-old G1P1 mother. She is breastfed every two hours for ten minutes on each breast. Her mother notes that the colostrum is now starting to change into breast milk. She stools after each feed, with the initially dark green stools are now changing to a yellowish color. She awakens approximately every three hours at night. Her mother is tired, but very happy, and says she is adjusting well. Her father, also at the appointment, says that he is excited to be able to feed AH once there is enough breast milk to pump and store in bottles.

Birth Hx: As noted above; uncomplicated NSVD, term

Prenatal Hx: Uncomplicated, no infections. Mother's prenatal labs: blood type O+, HbsAg negative, serum antibodies negative, PPD negative, gonorrhea/chlamydia negative, RPR non-reactive

Meds: None   **FHx:** Noncontributory

SHx: Lives with parents; both parents are employed, but taking maternity and paternity leave at this time; many family members (grandparents) and other social supports are involved

ROS: No fevers, activity consists of sleeping and eating, good bonding between infant and parents

VS: Stable

PE: Weight 3250 grams (birth weight 3290 grams). *Gen:* quiet, awake. *Skin:* jaundice to the face, no jaundice to trunk/abdomen/extremities, no bruising on skin, capillary refill time < 2 seconds. *HEENT:* scleral icterus present bilaterally, red reflex present bilaterally, anterior and posterior fontanels open/flat/soft, no cephalohematoma, mucous membranes moist. *CV:* no murmurs. *Chest:* CTA bilaterally. *Abdomen:* BS present, soft, no organomegaly. *Extremities:* no hip clicks. *Neuro:* present Moro reflex, symmetric suck/grasp/placing/rooting reflexes bilaterally. *Labs:* Blood type from cord blood O+.

THOUGHT QUESTIONS

- What type of jaundice does this patient have?
- How should this patient be managed?

AH has mild jaundice to the face only; history and examination is otherwise unremarkable. She is feeding well (current weight is not more than 10% less than birth weight), and excreting bilirubin via defecation. She is not dehydrated. Her jaundice is consistent with physiologic causes (that is, not due to pathologic processes), likely the delayed activity of hepatic glucuronyl transferase. Other causes of physiologic jaundice include decreased plasma clearance (poor feeding and decreased excretion) and hemoconcentration (dehydration). It can also be exacerbated in the setting of ABO incompatibility with a slight increase in hemolysis of the infant's erythrocytes due to maternal antibodies. Physiologic jaundice peaks at two to three days of life, disappearing in one week in term infants, and two weeks in preterm infants. This patient does not require any medical treatment or any phlebotomy. Patient education, reassurance, and encouragement should be given to the parents.

CASE CONTINUED

AH is taken home by her parents. They follow up a week later with complete resolution of her jaundice.

QUESTIONS

61. Which of the following is consistent with physiologic jaundice?
    A. Direct bilirubin level 1 mg/dl
    B. Schistocytes on a peripheral blood smear
    C. Cephalohematoma on examination
    D. Indirect bilirubin level of 20 mg/dl

62. Which infantile reflex may be normal when present at 10 months of age?
    A. Moro reflex
    B. Grasp (palmar) reflex
    C. Trunk incurvation (Galant's) reflex
    D. Positive Babinski response

63. Which of the following causes a direct hyperbilirubinemia?
    A. Delayed clamping of the umbilical cord at delivery
    B. Isoimmunization
    C. Vacuum-assisted vaginal delivery resulting in a cephalohematoma
    D. Biliary atresia

64. Kernicterus, a severe neurologic complication of hyperbilirubinemia, is characterized by bilirubin pigment deposition in the:
    A. Cerebral cortex
    B. Basal ganglia
    C. Hypothalamus
    D. Cerebellum

CASE 17 / SCHOOL FORMS

ID/CC: JA is a 2-year-old boy who is a new patient to the clinic, brought by his father who needs to have some forms filled out for preschool enrollment

HPI: The patient is in good health; father reports no problems. Development appears to be progressing normally according to the father who has two older children (ages 8 and 13). According to the father, the patient is playful, eats well, runs, jumps, and is very talkative. The preschool form requires a history and physical examination, as well as a list of immunizations received.

Birth Hx: Term NSVD to G1P1, no complications   **Meds:** None   **All:** NKDA

SHx: Parents divorced, custody recently awarded to father   **ROS:** Negative

DevHx: Passes Denver Developmental II – puts on own clothing, brushes teeth with some help, able to build a tower of six cubes, mostly understandable speech, names eight body parts, names five pictures, throws a ball overhand, jumps. *Immunizations:* Father does not know what immunizations the patient had in the past

PE: WNL

THOUGHT QUESTION

- What would entail an "up-to-date" immunization history for this patient?

The immunization schedule changes frequently; it is important for the family physician to be familiar with updates and changing guidelines/standard of care. Based on December 2001 recommended childhood immunization schedule by the AAFP, AAP, and ACIP, the child should have by this age:

- hepatitis B: three vaccinations (birth–2 months, 1–5 months, 6–18 months)
- diphtheria, tetanus, acellular pertussis: four vaccinations (2 months, 4 months, 6 months, 15–18 months)
- *Hemophilus influenzae* type b: four vaccinations (2 months, 4 months, 6 months, 12–15 months)
- inactivated polio: three vaccinations (2 months, 4 months, 6–18 months)
- pneumococcal conjugate: four vaccinations (2 months, 4 months, 6 months, 12–15 months)
- measles, mumps, rubella: one vaccination (12–15 months)
- varicella: one vaccination (12–18 months)

CASE CONTINUED

JA was born while his parents were stationed overseas and has not received the hepatitis B series. The first shot is administered and his parents are advised to follow up for the second shot in two to three months.

QUESTIONS

65. Which statement regarding vaccinations is false?
    A. Rotavirus vaccine is no longer recommended because it has been associated with intussusception
    B. Hepatitis A vaccine is recommended in areas with high risk for outbreaks
    C. Oral poliovirus is recommended for the fourth dose of polio vaccine
    D. The combined hepatitis B–*H. influenzae* type b vaccine may be used to decrease the number of administered shots

66. Which of the following statements regarding the MMR (measles, mumps, rubella) vaccine is false?
    A. It is formed of genetically engineered antigen designed to stimulate the immune response
    B. It should not be administered to pregnant teenagers
    C. A history of food allergies should be obtained prior to administration
    D. A history of allergies to medications should be obtained prior to administration

67. Which "immunization – type" pair is incorrectly matched?
    A. Varicella – live attenuated virus
    B. Pneumococcal – bacterial conjugate
    C. Diphtheria – bacterial toxoid
    D. Hepatitis B – live attenuated virus

68. All of the following are categories of development that are screened by the Denver Developmental II EXCEPT:
    A. Gross motor development
    B. Emotional development
    C. Personal-social development
    D. Language development

Vaccine ▼ / Age ►	Birth	1 mo	2 mos	4 mos	6 mos	12 mos	15 mos	18 mos	24 mos	4-6 yrs	11-12 yrs	13-18 yrs
						range of recommended ages		catch-up vaccination		preadolescent assessment		
Hepatitis B[1]	Hep B #1	only if mother HBsAg (-)								Hep B series		
			Hep B #2			Hep B #3						
Diphtheria, Tetanus, Pertussis[2]			DTaP	DTaP	DTaP		DTaP			DTaP	Td	
Haemophilus influenzae Type b[3]			Hib	Hib	Hib	Hib						
Inactivated Polio[4]			IPV	IPV		IPV				IPV		
Measles, Mumps, Rubella[5]						MMR #1				MMR #2	MMR #2	
Varicella[6]						Varicella				Varicella		
Pneumococcal[7]			PCV	PCV	PCV	PCV				PCV	PPV	
Hepatitis A[8]										Hepatitis A series		
Influenza[9]						Influenza (yearly)						

Vaccines below this line are for selected populations

This schedule indicates the recommended ages for routine administration of currently licensed childhood vaccines, as of December 1, 2001, for children through age 18 years. Any dose not given at the recommended age should be given at any subsequent visit when indicated and feasible. ▨ Indicates age groups that warrant special effort to administer those vaccines not previously given. Additional vaccines may be licensed and recommended during the year. Licensed combination vaccines may be used whenever any components of the combination are indicated and the vaccine's other components are not contraindicated. Providers should consult the manufacturers' package inserts for detailed recommendations.

1. Hepatitis B vaccine (Hep B). All infants should receive the first dose of hepatitis B vaccine soon after birth and before hospital discharge; the first dose may also be given by age 2 months if the infant's mother is HBsAg-negative. Only monovalent hepatitis B vaccine can be used for the birth dose. Monovalent or combination vaccine containing Hep B may be used to complete the series; four doses of vaccine may be administered if combination vaccine is used. The second dose should be given at least 4 weeks after the first dose, except for Hib-containing vaccine which cannot be administered before age 6 weeks. The third dose should be given at least 16 weeks after the first dose and at least 8 weeks after the second dose. The last dose in the vaccination series (third or fourth dose) should not be administered before age 6 months.

Infants born to HBsAg-positive mothers should receive hepatitis B vaccine and 0.5 mL hepatitis B immune globulin (HBIG) within 12 hours of birth at separate sites. The second dose is recommended at age 1-2 months and the vaccination series should be completed (third or fourth dose) at age 6 months.

Infants born to mothers whose HBsAg status is unknown should receive the first dose of the hepatitis B vaccine series within 12 hours of birth. Maternal blood should be drawn at the time of delivery to determine the mother's HBsAg status; if the HBsAg test is positive, the infant should receive HBIG as soon as possible (no later than age 1 week).

2. Diphtheria and tetanus toxoids and acellular pertussis vaccine (DTaP). The fourth dose of DTaP may be administered as early as age 12 months, provided 6 months have elapsed since the third dose and the child is unlikely to return at age 15-18 months. **Tetanus and diphtheria toxoids (Td)** is recommended at age 11-12 years if at least 5 years have elapsed since the last dose of tetanus and diphtheria toxoid-containing vaccine. Subsequent routine Td boosters are recommended every 10 years.

3. Haemophilus influenzae type b (Hib) conjugate vaccine. Three Hib conjugate vaccines are licensed for infant use. If PRP-OMP (PedvaxHIB® or ComVax® [Merck]) is administered at ages 2 and 4 months, a dose at age 6 months is not required. DTaP/Hib combination products should not be used for primary immunization in infants at age 2, 4 or 6 months, but can be used as boosters following any Hib vaccine.

4. Inactivated poliovirus vaccine (IPV). An all-IPV schedule is recommended for routine childhood poliovirus vaccination in the United States. All children should receive four doses of IPV at age 2 months, 4 months, 6-18 months, and 4-6 years.

5. Measles, mumps, and rubella vaccine (MMR). The second dose of MMR is recommended routinely at age 4-6 years but may be administered during any visit, provided at least 4 weeks have elapsed since the first dose and that both doses are administered beginning at or after age 12 months. Those who have not previously received the second dose should complete the schedule by the visit at 11-12 years.

6. Varicella vaccine. Varicella vaccine is recommended at any visit at or after age 12 months for susceptible children (i.e. those who lack a reliable history of chickenpox). Susceptible persons aged ≥13 years should receive two doses, given at least 4 weeks apart.

7. Pneumococcal vaccine. The heptavalent **pneumococcal conjugate vaccine (PCV)** is recommended for all children aged 2-23 months and for certain children aged 24-59 months. **Pneumococcal polysaccharide vaccine (PPV)** is recommended in addition to PCV for certain high-risk groups. See *MMWR* 2000;49(RR-9);1-37.

8. Hepatitis A vaccine. Hepatitis A vaccine is recommended for use in selected states and regions, and for certain high-risk groups; consult your local public health authority. See *MMWR* 1999;48(RR-12);1-37.

9. Influenza vaccine. Influenza vaccine is recommended annually for children age ≥ 6 months with certain risk factors (including but not limited to asthma, cardiac disease, sickle cell disease, HIV, and diabetes; see *MMWR* 2001;50(RR-4);1-44), and can be administered to all others wishing to obtain immunity. Children aged ≤12 years should receive vaccine in a dosage appropriate for their age (0.25 mL if age 6-35 months or 0.5 mL if aged ≥ 3 years). Children aged ≤ 8 years who are receiving influenza vaccine for the first time should receive two doses separated by at least 4 weeks.

For additional information about vaccines, vaccine supply, and contraindications for immunization, please visit the National Immunization Program Website at www.cdc.gov/nip or call the National Immunization Hotline at 800-232-2522 (English) or 800-232-0233 (Spanish).

Approved by the Advisory Committee on Immunization Practices (www.cdc.gov/nip/acip), the American Academy of Pediatrics (www.aap.org), and the American Academy of Family Physicians (www.aafp.org).

FIGURE 17 Child immunization schedule. (Source: www.cdc.gov.)

CASE 18 / SKIN LESION

ID/CC: MM comes in for evaluation of a mole on his back.

HPI: The patient is a 42-year-old Caucasian man who works in construction. His wife has been urging him to get the mole on his back removed for several years. She thinks it has become darker and bigger recently, although the patient can't see the mole himself. It is asymptomatic; however, last week it bled a little bit.

PMHx: Hypertension, hyperlipidemia   **PSHx:** None

Meds: Atorvastatin 20 mg per day, atenolol 50 mg per day, ASA 81 mg per day   **All:** NKDA

FHx: Father had an MI age 64, uncle had malignant melanoma

THOUGHT QUESTIONS
- What is the differential diagnosis of a pigmented skin lesion?
- What risk factors does this patient have for a malignant lesion?

There are two pigment-forming cells in the skin: the melanocyte and the nevus cell. Common pigmented growths include the following: freckle, lentigo, melasma, nevus, melanoma. Freckles are acquired before age 3 and darken with UV light exposure – they are therefore the result of increased *melanin* in the epidermis but a normal number of melanocytes. A lentigo is a brown macule that results from increased numbers of *melanocytes* and can be acquired at any age. Melasma is a patchy hyperpigmentation of the face, seen mostly in women and often as a result of pregnancy, birth control pills, or sun exposure. A nevus (mole) is a benign neoplasm of nevus cells; there are several different kinds: junctional, compound, Spitz, dysplastic, and blue. Nevi arise most commonly from birth to 40 years of age, and often regress later in life. Malignant melanoma is a neoplasm of melanocytes and nevus cells. Risk factors include sun exposure, family history of melanoma, immunosuppressive medications, presence of numerous nevi, and fair or freckled skin. Types of melanoma include superficial spreading, lentigo maligna, acral lentiginous, and nodular melanoma. Also keep in mind that although basal cell cancer is usually flesh-colored, occasional basal cell cancers are pigmented and resemble malignant melanoma.

VS: Temp 99°F BP 145/84 HR 66 RR 18

PE: Multiple small tan-colored macules on back, arms, legs. 9 × 5 mm irregularly shaped brown, speckled lesion that is slightly raised, left upper back. No axillary or groin lymphadenopathy

The patient states that his brother has had several "precancerous" lesions burned off in the office and asks if that is what you will do today. You explain that those sound like actinic keratoses and are different from the lesion he has.

THOUGHT QUESTIONS
- What is an actinic keratosis?
- Does it truly have malignant potential?

Actinic keratoses are very common lesions which are premalignant although the likelihood for malignant conversion into SCC is relatively low. AK begin as atypical squamous cells of the epidermis and tend to be sun-induced, thereby being most prominent on the face, scalp, hands, and forearms. The risk increases with age and is also higher in fair-skinned individuals. The lesions usually begin as a slightly rough raised area that over time develops a yellow crust and can bleed if trau-matized. Although the exact number of actinic keratoses that develop into SCC is unknown, it is thought that in an untreated patient SCC develops at a rate of 10–15% over a 10-year period (in the average affected patient presenting with seven or eight actinic keratoses).

Because of this small risk, it is better to treat AK as they develop. The treatment of choice for super-ficial AK is cryotherapy with liquid nitrogen, which is easily performed in the office. Other options include 5-FU, tretinoin plus 5-FU, glycolic acid peels, and masoprocol cream (a chemotherapeutic agent). For more indurated lesions or those with a thick crust a shave biopsy is probably the best.

THOUGHT QUESTION
- The patient looks concerned and says that his mother has "those keratosis things" all over her back –"looks like little pieces of tan silly putty stuck to her skin – but the doc said they were harmless and not to worry – could she get cancer?"

Seborrheic keratosis is different from *actinic* keratosis. Seborrheic keratoses are the most common benign skin cancer and grow within the epidermis. They can be flat, minimally raised, or more raised and are usually tan or brown colored, although occasionally they can be black-colored. The dark, irregular, irritated SKs can resemble malignant melanoma and need to be biopsied.

Because they are so superficial they look like they have been stuck onto the skin surface and can get chafed by clothing or when they are located in the intertriginous areas. They can itch too. Removal is only for cosmetic reasons, and is easily accomplished with cryotherapy or curettage.

THOUGHT QUESTION
- Another common, raised lesion is the wart – how are warts similar to seborrheic keratoses?

Warts are also benign epidermal neoplasms; however, they are caused by viral infection of the ker-atinocytes, mostly by HPV. Although SK appear in older patients, warts often occur in children and young adults. Many warts resolve spontaneously; many others will not disappear without treatment.

Warts can be treated with topical salicylic acid, liquid nitrogen cryotherapy, and electrocautery. Flat warts are harder to remove, and may require treatment with 5-FU (plus or minus tretinoin cream).

QUESTIONS

69. What is your next step?
    A. Referral to surgeon for evaluation
    B. Recheck in two to three months to see if lesion changes
    C. Biopsy today in office
    D. Topical hydroquinone to bleach the lesion

70. What kind of biopsy should be done?
    A. Shave biopsy
    B. Excisional biopsy
    C. Punch biopsy
    D. Incisional biopsy

71. What is the most common kind of skin cancer?
    A. Malignant melanoma
    B. Basal cell carcinoma
    C. Squamous cell carcinoma
    D. Kaposi's sarcoma

72. Match the skin cancer with the appropriate treatment
    A. Shave biopsy— melanoma
    B. Electrodessication and curettage—small squamous cell carcinoma
    C. Radiation—basal cell carcinoma
    D. Cryosurgery—invasive squamous cell carcinoma

ID/CC: TC is a 7-year-old boy who comes in for evaluation of a rash on his left abdomen.

HPI: The patient's mother reports that the rash has been present for two months, since the beginning of the summer. The rash is itchy and has spread slowly. The family has two dogs; however, the mother denies that the child has a history of allergies to pets or other environmental triggers. The mother denies using any new detergents, soap, creams, or underwear. She does now recall that the boy has a new pair of jeans with a lovely new belt from his Aunt Gertrude. She cannot remember if the jeans or the rash came first. On further questioning the mother states that she has some metal allergies, and can only wear 18 k gold earrings and bracelets.

PMHx: None   **PSHx:** Appendectomy age 6   **Meds:** Topical HC   **All:** NKDA

THOUGHT QUESTION
- What is the differential diagnosis of this rash? What workup is required?

Although there are many causes of a pruritic rash, the most common include fungal infection, eczema, psoriasis, scabies, and contact dermatitis. The physical exam is your most helpful diagnostic tool, aided by microscopic examination, and possibly a Wood's light exam, culture, or biopsy of the rash.

VS: Temp 98°F HR 90 RR 16

PE: *Skin:* 4-cm erythematous plaque with central clearing and a well-demarcated border in the left lower abdominal area. The border is scaly and elevated. A Wood's light exam does not fluoresce.

The mother is rushing to pick up her other son from school and does not want to stay to finish the appointment. You explain that you would like to do a scraping of the lesion to rule out a fungal cause, but she simply does not have the time. You look at the rash again and at the proximity to the belt buckle, which appears to be made of nickel, and decide that the rash is probably a contact dermatitis. You prescribe 0.5% betamethasone cream and tell them to get rid of the belt, preferably without offending Aunt Gertrude. A follow-up appointment is hastily made for three weeks later.

THOUGHT QUESTIONS
- What are the possible causes of contact dermatitis?
- What is the workup?

Contact dermatitis is an eczematous dermatitis caused by exposure to irritants or allergens. Irritant contact dermatitis is the most common, and occurs when the epidermis is damaged, as can happen with alkaline soaps, organic solvents, or long exposure to moisture such as with wet diapers or repetitive lip licking.

Allergic contact dermatitis is a delayed hypersensitivity reaction, and occurs in genetically predisposed people, often after several exposures to an antigenic substance. Common allergens include poison ivy and oak, hair tints, certain foods, latex, certain medications, rubber, nickel, cosmetics, deodorants, and jewelry. Nickel is the most common contact allergen, and is particularly common in women, probably because of frequent earring use.

Contact dermatitis is diagnosed with a careful history and PE. In cases of suspected allergic contact dermatitis, patch testing can be very useful. The patient avoids steroid creams and antihistamines for a week prior, then comes into the office for a battery of patch tests. Results are classified as:

negative reaction
    weak reaction: erythema
    strong reaction: erythema, edema, vesicles
    extreme reaction: spreading erythema and bullae, ulcerations

CASE CONTINUED

Two weeks later the patient and his mother return because the rash seems to be rapidly growing in size. The itching has improved, however. On exam the rash is now 6 cm in diameter and the borders are much less sharp and defined. The rash remains erythematous; however, within the rash are multiple red papules.

A scraping of material from the lesion is placed in a drop of KOH and examined under the microscope; hypha are seen.

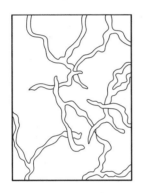

FIGURE 19 Hyphae under magnification. (Illustration by Electronic Illustrators Group.)

QUESTIONS

73. What is your diagnosis?
    A. Tinea corporis
    B. Eczema
    C. Atopic reaction to dogs
    D. Tinea capitis

74. What is the likely culprit?
    A. *Staph. epidermidis*
    B. Fleas
    C. Dermatophyte
    D. Scabies

75. What are the treatment options?
    A. Topical triamcinolone
    B. Topical miconazole
    C. Oral ketoconazole
    D. Calamine lotion and antihistamine as needed

76. What are considerations in prescribing oral antifungal agents?
    A. Diet
    B. Medication interactions
    C. Liver enzymes
    D. All of the above

ID/CC: A 41-year-old Caucasian woman comes in complaining of a rash on her face.

HPI: The red rash has been worsening over several months. The rash comes and goes on her face, and seems to get worse with sun exposure or after drinking hot tea. It is uncomfortable and stings or burns at times; it is also embarrassing and causes the patient significant distress. The patient denies any new makeup, although she has recently switched toothpastes. Occasionally she gets a headache and backache with the rash.

PMHx: Gastritis, depression   **PSHx:** Tonsillectomy age 5, breast augmentation 10 years ago

OBHx: Nulliparous   **GYNHx:** Normal Paps, LMP 25 days ago, IUD in place

Meds: Paroxetine 40 mg per day, lansoprazole 20 mg per day, $CaCO_3$ 500 mg twice a day   **All:** NKDA

SHx: Smokes one-half pack of cigarettes per day, no alcohol or drug use, works as an accountant

---

THOUGHT QUESTION

- What are the possible causes of the rash in this patient?

A waxing and waning erythematous rash in a 41-year-old woman is possibly secondary to acne vulgaris, rosacea, seborrheic dermatitis, steroid rosacea, perioral dermatitis, folliculitis, contact dermatitis, photosensitivity reactions, sarcoidosis, or systemic lupus erythematosus.

VS: Temp 97°F BP 104/77 HR 74 RR 12

PE: *Face:* multiple small inflammatory papules and pustules on forehead, cheeks, and chin on a background of erythema and telangiectases
Rest of skin exam WNL
Rest of PE WNL

THOUGHT QUESTIONS

- The patient is worried that she is going through puberty all over again and comments about how terrible it was to have acne as a teenager.
- Is this acne vulgaris?
- Is there more than one kind of acne?
- How is acne treated?

Acne vulgaris occurs when the sebaceous glands oversecrete sebum, usually in response to a change in the hormonal milieu. Sebum is irritating and comedogenic, resulting in follicular canal blockage. Concurrent infection with *Propionibacterium acnes*, an anaerobic diphtheroid, leads to inflammation and the formation of acne lesions.

Acne lesions are classified as inflammatory (papules, pustules, nodules) and noninflammatory (closed comedones and open comedones). Patients can have a combination of inflammatory and noninflammatory lesions, but usually have a preponderance of one, which facilitates the choice of therapeutic agents.

Treatments are as follows:

Topical: tretinoin gel/cream (increases cell turnover, prevents new comedones)
adapalene cream
microsphere tretinoin
tazarotene cream
azelaic acid
benzoyl peroxide (antibacterial, drying)
antibiotics (tetracycline, clindamycin, erythromycin)

Oral: antibiotics (tetracycline, erythromycin, doxycycline, clindamycin, ampicillin, cephalexin,
trimethoprim/sulfamethoxasole, azithromycin)
isotretinoin (reduces sebum excretion, follicular keratinization, antibacterial)
OCPs

The treatment of choice for noninflammatory acne is tretinoin cream. Adapalene and microsphere tretinoin work in the same way but are less irritating and cause less sun sensitivity. Tazarotene is also a vitamin A analog but is more irritating and is best for patients with very oily skin.

Isotretinoin pills are best reserved for severe inflammatory and cystic acne, patients who scar easily, patients for whom even mild acne causes severe depression or dysmorphic disorders, patients with atypical acne, and patients who are unresponsive to conventional treatments. The acne usually clears completely in 85% of patients within four months; 39% relapse after the isotretinoin is withdrawn with 23% requiring oral antibiotic therapy and 16% requiring another course of isotretinoin.

The most common side effect is cheilitis, which is almost universal and treated by applying emollients. Cheilitis is described as dryness and a burning sensation at the corners of the mouth; the skin there wrinkles and can even fissure. Other side effects include decreased bone density, increased LFTs, and increased TGs. Isotretinoin is a powerful teratogen and therefore all women of childbearing age on the medicine must be on two forms of birth control and get a pregnancy test before starting. While on the medicine patients should have monthly CBC, TG, and LFTs.

For patients with "ice-pick scarring" treatment options include scar revision, dermabrasion, and laser resurfacing.

Other kinds of acne include gram-negative acne, neonatal acne, occupational acne, acne mechanica, acne cosmetica, and excoriated acne secondary to excessive traumatic picking of the lesions.

QUESTIONS

77. You feel that the H&P are consistent with rosacea, which can be complicated by all of the following EXCEPT:
    A. Rhinophyma
    B. Eye involvement
    C. Folliculitis
    D. Sinusitis

78. Appropriate treatment involves:
    A. Benzoyl peroxide
    B. Astringents
    C. Intravenous antibiotics
    D. Topical antibiotics

79. The patient returns for her follow-up visit, visibly pleased with her improvement. Her 22-year-old niece accompanies her, hoping for similar treatment and improvement for her facial rash, which they assume may be rosacea as well. She has hypopigmented and pink macules with some scaling on the forehead, eyebrows, and nasolabial folds; she also has some dandruff. Her most likely diagnosis is:
    A. Seborrheic dermatitis
    B. Psoriasis
    C. Atopic dermatitis
    D. Rosacea

80. Treatment options include the following EXCEPT:
    A. Steroid shampoo
    B. Antifungal shampoo
    C. Selenium shampoo
    D. Antibiotic shampoo

CASE 21 / INGUINAL MASS

ID/CC: IH is a 24-year-old man coming in for evaluation of a groin mass.

HPI: The patient describes a mass present in his right groin for six months. It started out as a small and asymptomatic mass, but has been slowly growing in size and discomfort. It is not present when the patient lies in bed at night. He denies any vomiting or change in bowel habits.

PMHx: None **PSHx:** None **Meds:** Tylenol, Ibuprofen as needed **All:** NKDA

THOUGHT QUESTION
- What is the differential diagnosis of a groin mass?

The differential diagnosis of a groin mass includes:

- enlarged inguinal lymph node: more lateral in location and distal to groin crease, can be bilateral, no change in size with Valsalva, usually multiple
- a lipoma: can be palpated to be separate from underlying fascia and only in subcutaneous tissue
- a hydrocele of the spermatic cord: mass is primarily scrotal in position, transilluminates well
- a saphenous vein varix: softer than a hernia, bluish color underneath the skin
- a psoas muscle abscess: less well-defined than a hernia, lateral to the femoral artery
- hernia: see below

The physical exam serves to differentiate herniation from other causes of inguinal swelling or pain. The most likely diagnosis in this patient is a hernia.

CASE CONTINUED

VS: Temp 97°F BP 132/78 HR 82 RR 12

PE: Well-appearing man in no acute distress. *Lungs:* CTA. *CV:* RRR. Abdomen soft, nontender, nondistended, no hepatosplenomegaly. In supine position no inguinal masses palpated. In standing position with Valsalva right 2 to 3 cm slightly tender inguinal mass palpated, with abdominal muscle relaxation you are able to gently reduce the size of the mass until it is barely palpable.

THOUGHT QUESTION
- The patient's brother had a left inguinal herniorrhaphy at age 6 months and the patient wonders whether his hernia is genetic. Are pediatric and adult hernias exactly the same?

The etiology and differential diagnosis are similar, and indirect inguinal hernias are the most common kind of hernia in both adults and children. However, in adults 50% of all hernias are indirect, whereas in children 99% are indirect.

Inguinal hernias are broadly classified as direct or indirect, designations that refer to the relation of the herniation to the inferior epigastric arteries on the abdominal wall and the Hesselbach's triangle.

Indirect inguinal hernias pass through the internal abdominal inguinal ring along the spermatic cord, through the inguinal canal, and exit through the external inguinal ring. In direct inguinal hernias the abdominal contents pass through the posterior inguinal wall in Hesselbach's triangle. An indirect hernia passes lateral to the inferior epigastric vessels and thus is outside of Hesselbach's triangle, while a direct hernia is medial to the epigastric vessels and therefore within the confines of this space. An indirect hernia is generally believed to have a congenital component, whereas direct inguinal hernias are acquired by deficiencies of the transversus abdominus muscle, which makes up the floor of the inguinal canal.

Inguinal hernias are the most common surgical condition in children, and the boy to girl ratio is 4:1. 50% present before age 1, and 60% are on the right side, 30% are on the left side, and 10% are bilateral. Hernias occur in 10 to 20 infants per 1000 live births; the prevalence among preemies verges on 30%.

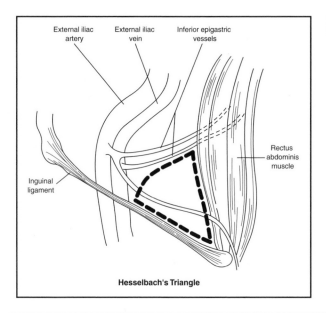

FIGURE 21 Hesselbach's triangle. (Illustration by Electronic Illustrators Group.)

Although acquired defects in the transversalis fascia account for a good portion of hernias in adults, congenital defects are largely responsible for hernias in infants. The processus vaginalis is a diverticular protrusion of the peritoneum that forms ventral to the gubernaculum, and herniates through the abdominal wall into the inguinal canal in the third trimester. During the last few weeks of gestation, the layers of the processus vaginalis normally fuse together and obliterate the entrance to the inguinal canal. Failure of the obliteration results in an inguinal hernia.

The treatment of choice in infants is repair. Most pediatric surgeons recommend bilateral inguinal exploration at the time of surgery in all boys younger than 1 year old, all girls younger than 2 years old, and all patients with conditions associated with increased risks of hernia.

THOUGHT QUESTION
• Are all surgical hernia repairs the same?

Answer: Inguinal hernias can be repaired open or laparoscopically. Open surgical repairs have been the treatment of choice until very recently, in which the surgeon sutures the conjoined tendon of the transversus abdominis together with the internal oblique muscles and the inguinal ligament. Most repairs now include mesh reinforcement of the inguinal floor for improved strength of the repair. Open repairs can be done with general or local anesthesia. Laparoscopic repairs require general anesthesia.

QUESTIONS

81. What kind of hernia is most probable in this young male patient with the above PE findings?
    A. Ventral
    B. Femoral
    C. Indirect inguinal
    D. Direct inguinal

82. Based on the patient's H&P you decide the hernia is:
    A. Reducible
    B. Incarcerated
    C. Strangulated
    D. None of the above

83. Based on your tentative diagnosis you next order:
    A. An ultrasound
    B. A surgery consult
    C. An MRI
    D. CBC, ESR

84. The patient asks about his treatment options. You inform him that
    A. He needs to go to the ER for immediate admission and surgery
    B. Surgery will be scheduled electively
    C. The surgery requires general anesthesia
    D. After surgical repair his risk for hernia recurrence is 15–20%

ID/CC: It is 10 p.m. and you are called in to the ER to see a patient of yours complaining of abdominal pain. The ER doc thinks it may be appendicitis.

HPI: CC is a 33-year-old G3P3 who began to experience right-sided abdominal pain this evening after dinner. She describes the pain as rather rapid in onset, and cannot localize it well other than stating it is on her right side. She vomited once, and feels ill. The pain is constant and seems to be worsening. She had diarrhea twice today, and denies dysuria or back pain.

She has never had abdominal pain like this before and rates it 8/10. She ate tamales and rice at dinner and states that she's often had this meal in the past without problems.

THOUGHT QUESTION
- As you hang up the phone you remember that your professors in medical school always harped on the importance of the history in diagnosing abdominal pain. What did they mean?

The history in a patient with abdominal pain divulges a lot:

- Chronology: —rapid onset: cholecystitis, pancreatitis, perforated ulcer, mesenteric infarction, AAA rupture, ruptured ectopic pregnancy
  —gradual onset: appendicitis, diverticulitis, SBO, gastroenteritis, PID
  —progression: gastroenteritis will resolve, appendicitis will progress, etc.
- Location: —periumbilical: appendicitis, SBO, mesenteric infarction, gastroenteritis
  —RLQ: appendicitis, ovarian torsion, TOA, ruptured ectopic
  —RUQ: cholecystitis, hepatitis
  —epigastric, back: pancreatitis, AAA, perforated peptic ulcer
  —LLQ, pelvic: diverticulitis, PID, ectopic pregnancy
- Character: —diffuse: appendicitis, perforated peptic ulcer, SBO, mesenteric infarction, ruptured AAA, gastroenteritis
  —localized: appendicitis (late), cholecystitis, pancreatitis, diverticulitis, PID
- Aggravating and relieving factors: position, eating, time of day, etc.
- ROS

CASE CONTINUED

PMHx: Nephrolithiasis 3 years ago   **PSHx:** C/S × 1

OBHx: C/S 10 years ago, NSVD/successful VBAC 8 and 5 years ago

GYNHx: No STDs, no Paps for two years but previously normal   **Meds:** Tamoxifen prophylaxis

All: PCN → rash   **FHx:** DM II, obesity, HTN, breast CA (mother and half-sister)

THOUGHT QUESTIONS
- What is the differential diagnosis of her abdominal pain?
- As you drive to the hospital you consider appendicitis. Is her presentation really classic for appendicitis?

Common causes of right-sided abdominal pain include appendicitis, ovarian torsion or ruptured cyst, ectopic pregnancy, PID/TOA, cholecystitis, cecal diverticulitis, acute gastroenteritis, small bowel obstruction, and pancreatitis.

Acute unruptured appendicitis classically presents with prodromal symptoms of anorexia, nausea, and vague periumbilical pain which slowly migrates to the right lower quadrant. Patients often have a low-grade temperature and mild leukocytosis, and on exam demonstrate rebound and tenderness to palpation of the right lower quadrant. However, the classic presentation occurs in only 50% of patients:

TABLE 22. Symptoms of Acute Unruptured Appendicitis	
SYMPTOMS	FREQUENCY
Abdominal pain	100%
Anorexia	100%
Nausea	90%
Vomiting	75%
Pain migration	50%

VS: Temp 99°F BP 100/60 HR 103 RR 20

PE: Weight 170 lbs, Height 5'3". Lungs CTA, CV ST. *Abdomen:* soft, tender to palpation RUQ w/o HSM (hepatosplenomegaly), moderate tenderness epigastric area, less tenderness RLQ, no rebound or guarding. No CVAT (costovertebral angle tenderness). *BME:* no CMT (cervical motion tenderness), uterus midline and nontender, no adnexal masses or tenderness, no discharge. *DRE:* NST (normal sphincter tone), guaiac-negative brown stool, no masses.

Labs: WBC 14.7, Hb 12.3, PLT 303, Neutrophils 85, Lymph 11, Mono 4, Chem-7 WNL. *Urinalysis:* normal.

QUESTIONS

85. You feel that the H&P are not necessarily consistent with appendicitis, and instead consider cholecystitis. What risk factors does the patient have for gallbladder disease?
    A. History of nephrolithiasis
    B. Prior abdominal surgery
    C. Tamoxifen
    D. Obesity

86. You order LFTs and an abdominal ultrasound. Bilirubin is 1.8, AST is 94, ALT is 65, alk phos is 246. The ultrasound demonstrates gallstones with a thickened gallbladder wall, a positive Murphy's sign (the sudden, involuntary arrest of inspiration when the examiner palpates the RUQ), and a normal common bile duct. The appendix is noted to be 5 mm in diameter. You diagnose the patient with:
    A. Acute cholecystitis
    B. Acute appendicitis
    C. Choledocholithiasis
    D. Cholangitis

87. Your next step is:
    A. IVF, pain medications, discharged home when stable and follow-up outpatient
    B. Lap cholecystectomy within 24–48 hours
    C. ERCP
    D. Open cholecystectomy

88. Possible complications of gallstones include:
    A. Small bowel obstruction
    B. Gallbladder cancer
    C. Hepatitis B
    D. Acute gastritis

ID/CC: A 28-year-old African-American man comes to your drop-in acute care clinic complaining of an unbearable headache.

HPI: LJ is a previously healthy man who describes having a severe right-sided headache for the past five nights. The headache starts after he lies down and is intermittent, but definitely worse at night. He feels like he is unable to sleep. He describes the pain as stabbing; it makes his eyes water. He fears that he has high blood pressure like his brother.

PMHx: One compound tibia fracture at age 12   **Meds:** Occasional acetaminophen

All: NKDA   **FHx:** Brother with HTN

THOUGHT QUESTIONS

- What parts of his history need to be clarified?
- What are the different classifications and types of headaches?

Headaches are one of the most common complaints presented to primary care physicians. Therefore, a systematic approach will help simplify the visit. Headaches can be divided into acute and chronic types (although every chronic type will have an initial presentation). Characteristics of an acute (<24 hour) headache may include: sudden onset, severe pain, persistent nature. The history should focus on associated symptoms of fever, history of trauma, neck stiffness, neurological problems, circumstances when it started, nausea/vomiting, eye pain or blurred vision. Recurrent or persistent headaches, such as the one presented above, can often be diagnosed by history alone. Timing of headache and associated symptoms are often diagnostic; location, intensity, and quality of headache can also be helpful. Key questions include: Do you have symptom-free periods? How long do the headaches last? Do medicines relieve the pain? Do you have a premonition or aura before the headache starts? As with any somatic complaint, you should obtain a full social history, history of substance use, and depression screening. Caffeine and alcohol intake, erratic sleep patterns, and MSG (the food additive) increase the risk of headache.

TABLE 23. Etiologies of Headaches	
ETIOLOGIES OF ACUTE HEADACHE	**ETIOLOGIES OF PERSISTENT OR RECURRENT CHRONIC HEADACHE**
viral illness, CO poisoning, hypoglycemia, acute sinusitis, glaucoma, cerebral or intracranial hemorrhage, and meningitis	mass lesion (including AVM), medication side effect, TMJ/bruxism, substance abuse, hypertension, tension-type headache, migraine with or without aura, cluster headache, cervical radiculopathy, and temporal arteritis

CASE CONTINUED

LJ denies regular substance use. He drinks one cup of regular coffee per day and smokes occasional marijuana. His headache pain lasts about two to three hours at a time, at least two times during the night. During the day he feels tired and occasionally has a throbbing feeling near his right eye. Last night during his most severe episode, his right eye was red and he felt like his right cheek was sweating. The pain was so severe he sat upright and rocked for two hours; 500 mg of acetaminophen did nothing to relieve the pain. He currently has no pain.

VS: BP 125/75 HR 75 RR 16, afebrile

PE: Tired-appearing man, NAD. *HEENT:* PERRLA, EOMI, disc margins sharp. No frontal or maxillary TTP, no scalp or forehead TTP. TMJ nontender. *Neck:* supple, no meningismus, negative Sperling's (test for cervical stenosis). *CV/Pulm:* normal. *Abdomen:* normal. *Extremities:* no C/C/E. *Neuro:* Alert and oriented. CN II-XII grossly intact. Sensation/ motor intact. Negative Romberg. Normal heel-toe gait. Reflexes 2+ throughout.

THOUGHT QUESTIONS
- What is your diagnosis for this patient?
- What is the typical pattern for this diagnosis?
- What are treatment options?

This patient presents with recent onset cluster headache. It is most common in middle-age men and usually occurs in cycles lasting several weeks to months. It is unilateral (although it may switch sides between episodes) and is severe, retro-ocular, and recurrent. Typically the pain occurs at night and lasts 15 minutes to 3 hours. It may be associated with lacrimation and nasal congestion on the ipsilateral side. Attacks may be provoked by alcohol, smoking, or nitroglycerine use. Increased cerebral blood flow to the affected side with partial compression of the sympathetic plexus may cause the constellation of symptoms. Ibuprofen is successful in relieving pain in a small percentage of patients. Abortive therapy includes: ergotamine suppositories once at bedtime, dihydroergotamine IM, sumitriptan subcutaneous or by mouth, or high-flow inhaled O_2 for 10 minutes (ideal in the ER for diagnostic purposes). Prednisone taper over two weeks can also be used for prolonged symptoms. Prophylactic therapy may include calcium-channel blockers for patients with severe episodes.

CASE CONTINUED

You prescribe LJ with a small supply of sumitriptan. Phone follow-up one week later reveals that he has taken three doses since his visit and has been symptom-free for the past four days.

QUESTIONS

89. Which of the following signs or symptoms is inconsistent with migraine headache?
    A. Transient aphasia
    B. Confusion, poor memory, loss of concentration
    C. Vomiting
    D. Auras that last for more than 24 hours

90. Which of the following options for prophylaxis of migraine headache would not be appropriate?
    A. Beta-blockers
    B. Tricyclic antidepressants
    C. Progesterone supplementation
    D. Naproxen

91. Cranial arteritis is characterized by all of the following except:
    A. It usually affects patients over age 50
    B. The inflamed temporal artery is always tender
    C. Blindness is the most serious complication
    D. This arteritis affects medium and large arteries

92. Chronic tension-type headaches are:
    A. Almost always unilateral
    B. Restricted to hours of waking when stress is most apparent
    C. Characterized by tenderness to palpation of the muscles of the head and neck
    D. Best treated by regular, acute-relief medications

ID/CC: A 38-year-old Filipino woman presents to your urgent care clinic saying that the right side of her mouth is drooping.

HPI: LP is an otherwise healthy woman who last saw a doctor $1^1/_2$ years ago for health care maintenance. She has been feeling a little tired recently and last night did not sleep too well. This morning when she awoke she felt burning right ear pain; when she went to the bathroom she noticed in the mirror that the right side of her mouth was drooping and she couldn't make her smile equal on both sides. Her right eyelid also felt like it was stuck open. She is very worried: "Am I having a stroke?" No complaint of fever, chills, nausea, vomiting, or headache. She is able to walk, think, and move normally. No visual complaints.

ROS: LMP 6 weeks ago, normal; using rhythm method of contraception   **PMHx:** None

Meds: Occasional ibuprofen   **All:** NKDA   **FHx:** Sister with asthma

VS: BP 115/76 HR 85 RR 16; afebrile, walking without difficulty

PE: *HEENT:* Right nasolabial fold droop. PERRLA, EOMI. Right forehead is smooth. TMs bilaterally pearly with no effusion; canals normal-appearing. No parotid masses. *Neuro:* Alert and oriented, CN II-XII on left intact. On right, dense VIIth nerve weakness including the forehead and slightly decreased corneal reflex. Other right CN intact. Peripheral reflexes normal. Gait normal, Romberg negative. *Skin:* No vesicles, erythema, or induration around right face or ear.

THOUGHT QUESTIONS
- What is the differential diagnosis for this patient?
- What key parts of the history and physical point to the diagnosis?
- What studies need to be done?
- What symptoms would trigger an MRI?

This patient presents with a unilateral facial palsy. By far the most common cause is Bell's palsy, an idiopathic unilateral acute peripheral nerve palsy, which causes more than 80% of facial palsies. First, it is necessary to demonstrate that it is not a central lesion, which would spare the upper face distribution.

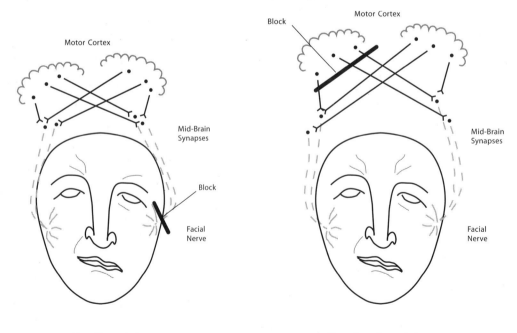

Lower Motor Neuron Lesion =
Entire Side Affected

Upper Motor Neuron Lesion =
Forehead spared 2° some ipsilateral ennervation

FIGURE 24 Anatomy of facial nerve distribution and examples of lesions. (Illustration by Shawn Girsberger, Graphic Design.)

In this patient, the right forehead is equally affected, so it is clearly a peripheral palsy. Other causes of peripheral facial palsy include trauma (fracture of the temporal bone), bacterial infection, sarcoid, Guillain-Barre' syndrome, chilling of the face, and tumor (acoustic neuroma, neurofibroma, cholesteotoma, and others). This patient's acute onset, lack of other symptoms, and benign physical exam all point to Bell's palsy. In the uncomplicated patient with Bell's palsy, no additional tests need to be done. A radiographic study would be indicated if a mass is suspected, or if the patient has a persistent or atypical case. However, in this patient with LMP six weeks prior, a urine pregnancy test should be performed. Bell's palsy is more common in pregnancy, and also in hypothyroidism and diabetes.

CASE CONTINUED

Her urine pregnancy test is negative. You discuss your diagnosis with your patient. She is initially very alarmed, but then reassured as she learns more information. You prescribe two medicines and arrange to see her again in one week. You also give her a patient education manual to share with her family.

QUESTIONS

93. What percentage of patients with Bell's palsy achieve full spontaneous recovery?
    A. 95%
    B. 50%
    C. 30%
    D. 70%

94. What medicines may have benefit acutely in treating Bell's palsy?
    A. Prednisone
    B. Acyclovir
    C. Natural tears
    D. None of the above
    E. All of the above

95. Which muscle is implicated in the most serious consequence of Bell's palsy?
    A. Orbicularis oculi
    B. Masseter
    C. Platysma
    D. Frontalis

96. What is the incidence of Bell's palsy in the general population?
    A. 1/1000 people per year
    B. 1/65 people per lifetime
    C. 1/250 people per lifetime
    D. 1/100 women per lifetime; 1/1000 men per lifetime

ID/CC: WT is a 64-year-old Caucasian male who presents to the acute care clinic complaining of a headache over the last four hours.

HPI: WT tells you that his headache started like his normal migraine initially, but became much more severe in the past few hours. He has blurry vision, different from the normal auras he usually gets with the migraines. He had emesis twice in the past hour, and wants an antiemetic/analgesic injection for what he believes is a more severe migraine. No weakness or numbness. He notes a cold in the past week with nasal congestion, sore throat, and a cough, for which he has been taking OTC decongestants and cough syrup. No CP/SOB.

PMHx: Migraine headaches, HTN, chronic renal insufficiency with proteinuria and a baseline creatinine of 2.0, DM 2, carpal tunnel syndrome.

Meds: The patient tells you his prescription medications, but says he ran out one week ago. HCTZ 25 mg once a day, clonidine 0.1 mg once a day, metformin 500 mg three times a day with meals, acetaminophen with codeine for migraine headaches, OTC pseudoephedrine 60 mg four times a day, OTC cough syrup.

All: NKDA

FHx: Father and mother both had HTN. Mother with ESRD secondary to DM 2 and HTN, died at 65 years old. Father with MI, died at 59 years old.

SHx: Retired tour bus driver, lives alone, divorced without any children

Habits: Smokes one-half pack of cigarettes per day for 40 years, social alcohol, occasional cocaine, occasional cannabis

ROS: Noted above in the HPI, otherwise negative   **VS:** Afebrile BP 254/160 HR 96 RR 18 99% RA

PE: *Gen:* in discomfort, full sentences. *HEENT:* NC/AT, PERRLA, EOMI, bilateral papilledema on ophthalmoscopic examination, no retinal hemorrhages, OP clear, tongue midline. *Neck:* no bruits, no JVD. *CV:* RRR no murmurs, normal S1, S2. *Chest:* CTA bilaterally. *Abd:* benign. *Neuro:* oriented × 3, nonfocal except for papilledema. *Urine dipstick:* + blood/protein, otherwise negative. *EKG:* NSR at 96, no ST segment changes or abnormal T waves

---

THOUGHT QUESTION
- What is the differential diagnosis?

The differential includes hypertensive emergency, subarachnoid hemorrhage, and stroke. Given WT's presentation with significantly elevated blood pressures, papilledema, and hematuria, a hypertensive emergency is the most likely diagnosis. If WT had focal neurologic deficits, stroke would be the leading diagnosis. If WT presented with nuchal rigidity, a subarachnoid hemorrhage would be more probable. If stroke or SAH were more concerning, a head CT followed by a lumbar puncture would be necessary diagnostic measures.

CASE CONTINUED

The patient is admitted to the hospital for a hypertensive emergency. He was treated appropriately, and discharged with followup with his PMD in one week. His antihypertensive regiment was also adjusted while he was hospitalized.

THOUGHT QUESTION
- What is a hypertensive emergency?

A hypertensive emergency occurs with severely elevated blood pressures with signs and symptoms of end-organ damage (brain, heart, kidneys). The blood pressure must be reduced within one hour to reduce serious morbidity or death. There is no specific blood pressure value which defines a hypertensive emergency; it is the organ damage that results from the elevated blood pressures that defines an emergency.

TABLE 25. Organ System Damage

ORGAN SYSTEM	EVIDENCE OF END-ORGAN DAMAGE
Neurologic	Encephalopathy, headache, irritability, altered mental status, papilledema, intracranial hemorrhage
Cardiovascular	Unstable angina, pulmonary edema, myocardial infarction, aortic dissection
Renal	Hematuria, proteinuria, progressive renal dysfunction

A hypertensive urgency occurs with significantly elevated blood pressures without evidence of end organ damage. These blood pressures can be reduced over the course of a few hours, and rarely require parenteral therapy.

The terms "malignant hypertension," "hypertensive crisis," and "accelerated hypertension" are obsolete.

QUESTIONS

97. Which antihypertensive medication should be first-line therapy in this patient?
    A. Angiotensin-converting enzyme inhibitor
    B. Angiotensin receptor blocker
    C. Potassium-sparing diuretic
    D. Calcium channel blocker

98. Which of the following did not contribute to the patient's hypertensive emergency?
    A. Noncompliance with prescription medications
    B. Cocaine inhalation
    C. Use of over-the-counter decongestant and cough syrup
    D. Cannabis inhalation

99. Which of the following images represents this patient's ophthalmoscopic examination?
    A. Figure 25a

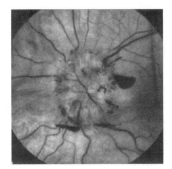

FIGURE 25a Funduscopic examination. (Image courtesy of Arthur D. Fu, MD.)

    B. Figure 25b

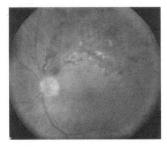

FIGURE 25b Funduscopic examination. (Image courtesy of Arthur D. Fu, MD.)

    C. Figure 25c

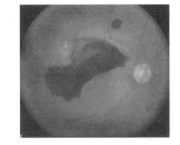

FIGURE 25c Funduscopic examination. (Image courtesy of Arthur D. Fu, MD.)

    D. Figure 25d

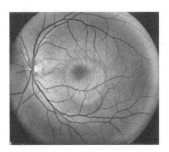

FIGURE 25d Funduscopic examination. (Image courtesy of Arthur D. Fu, MD.)

100. Which of the following statements is true regarding the treatment of a hypertensive emergency?
    A. The blood pressure should immediately be reduced to normal values
    B. Oral anti-hypertensives are just as effective as parenteral therapy
    C. Intravenous nitroprusside can be easily titrated to a goal blood pressure, and yields immediate anti-hypertensive effect
    D. Treatment of a hypertensive emergency is warranted only if the blood pressure is >250/150

ID/CC: A 42-year-old Caucasian woman comes to her regular appointment and complains that she has been feeling dizzy.

HPI: FS is well-known to you; you see her approximately every six months. Her last visit had focused mostly on perimenopausal issues and she had been adjusting to her only child going to college. She says that since then she has been having "dizzy spells," sometimes every day, sometimes every five to seven days. She describes feeling sweaty and light-headed, then having to sit or lie down for about 10 minutes before she feels better. She has not fainted that she knows of. She is now afraid this will happen when she is driving.

PMHx: 1. Perimenopausal; occasional hot flashes, LMP four months ago. 2. Plantar fasciitis. 3. Benign breast biopsy two years prior. 4. Lipids one year ago: total 180, HDL 60, LDL 95

Meds: 1. Soy flour for menopausal symptoms. 2. Multivitamin

All: PCN causes hives   **FHx:** Non-contributory

SHx: As above, lives alone; works as assistant in accounting firm.

Habits: One cup coffee in the morning, no other caffeine. No cigarettes, three to four glasses of wine a week; no other recreational drugs.

THOUGHT QUESTIONS
- What is the differential diagnosis for this type of problem?
- What questions could you ask our patient to help clarify what's been going on?

This differential is huge! However, "dizziness" is a very common complaint in primary care. Dizziness should first be divided into the two major categories: vertigo—head sensation of abnormal movement; and light-headedness—a sense of faintness from insufficient cerebral perfusion or severe metabolic abnormality.

TABLE 26. Causes of Dizziness by Type of Dizziness Experienced

VERTIGO		
PERIPHERAL LESION	**CENTRAL LESION**	**LIGHT-HEADEDNESS OR NEAR-SYNCOPE**
Benign positional vertigo (BPV), head trauma, Meniere's disease, acute labyrinthitis, ototoxins, and acoustic neuroma	Multiple sclerosis, vertebrobasilar insufficiency, sedatives, anticonvulsants	Neurocardiogenic syncope, autonomic insufficiency, carotid sinus hypersensitivity, posttussive or postmicturition syncope, cerebrovascular disease, subclavian steal, effort syncope (valvular disease), dysrhythmias, seizures, and metabolic abnormality,

Dysequilibrium (less common) is a sensation of abnormal balance that starts in the feet. Also, psychiatric problems can cause a feeling of fogginess or light-headedness. Extreme hyperventilation causes metabolic alkalosis which can then cause light-headedness or vertigo.

Important questions to ask regarding vertigo are, "Do you see things spinning or moving? Do you have ringing or hearing loss in your ears (labyrinthitis or Meniere's)? Are your symptoms triggered by a certain movement or position (BPV)? Do you have pressure in your ears (Meniere's)? Are your symptoms getting worse (acoustic neuroma)?" And, for light-headedness, "Are your symptoms brought on with exercise, with change of position, or after you cough or use the rest room? Have you ever felt palpitations or chest pain with symptoms (cardiac disease)? Have you ever had a seizure or lost bowel or bladder control? Do you have premonitory symptoms?"

CASE CONTINUED

Your patient is able to provide a detailed history. She denies any vertiginous symptoms. She does have a prodrome: feeling dizzy, light-headed, and slightly nauseated. She denies chest pain or palpitations. She hasn't noticed particular actions or positions that bring it on. She has had several witnessed events at work; co-workers noted that she looked pale and unwell, but never had tonic-clonic movements. She has never had residual neurologic problems.

VS: BP 120/75 HR 85 RR 16 O_2 Saturation 99% on RA five-minute orthostatics: no significant change.

PE: *HEENT:* atraumatic, PERRLA, EOMI. *Neck:* supple, no LAN. Carotid pulses with normal upstroke bilaterally, no bruit. *CV:* RRR, no M/R/G, normal PMI. *Pulmonary:* CTA. *Extremities:* no C/C/E. *Neuro:* Reflexes 2+ throughout, Romberg –, strength, sensation, gait intact.

THOUGHT QUESTION
- What two tests are indicated now?

Random laboratory studies searching for a cause of near-syncope in an otherwise healthy patient usually do not find any useful information. This patient needs an EKG on the basis of age to look for ischemic change, conduction system abnormality, or arrhythmia. On the basis of history, she then needs upright tilt-testing.

CASE CONTINUED

She has a positive tilt-test for neurocardiogenic disease and is started on a therapeutic medicine. Two months later she hasn't had any attacks and is feeling much better.

QUESTIONS

101. What is the medication of choice for neurocardiogenic syncope?
    A. Benzodiazepine
    B. Beta blocker
    C. SSRI
    D. Nitroglycerine

102. The one-year mortality risk for cardiac syncope is _____ that for unexplained or non-cardiac syncope.
    A. The same as
    B. Twice
    C. Three times
    D. Four times

103. All of the following tests may be indicated to evaluate a suspected cardiac origin of syncope except:
    A. Echocardiogram
    B. Holter monitor
    C. Exercise stress test
    D. V/Q scan

104. A 68-year-old man complains of seeing the room spin whenever he looks quickly to the left. It lasts for several minutes, then goes away on its own. In the absence of other symptoms, the most likely diagnosis is:
    A. Meniere's disease
    B. Acoustic neuroma
    C. Acute labyrinthitis
    D. Benign positional vertigo

ID/CC: A 62-year-old Latina woman presents to you for a new patient appointment. She complains of chest pain that she has noticed for about six months when walking up hills.

HPI: GM is a pleasant, obese woman accompanied by her daughter. She describes the pain as a burning/pressure in the left side of her chest that comes on only when walking up the steepest hills near her apartment. It goes away within two to five minutes of rest. She does feel short of breath "because I'm walking up a hill." She has no symptoms of palpitations, sweating, nausea, or vomiting. She gets the chest pain one or two times per week, never at rest. She denies any chest pain currently. Her normal exercise tolerance is about one-half mile on flat surfaces.

PMHx: Unknown; she denies any problems.   **Meds:** Occasional herbal remedy.   **All:** NKDA

FHx: Father died of "heart problem" at age 55; mother has DM, lives in Guatemala. Siblings are all healthy to her knowledge.

SHx: Just moved here two months ago from Guatemala, living with daughter. Helps to care for grandchildren. Smokes one to two cigars per day. No alcohol or other drugs.

ROS: Urinates three times per night. Drinking more water since moving to the United States.

VS: BP 145/90 HR 82 NAD

PE: *Neck:* no JVD. *CV:* RRR. No M/R/G; no chest wall TTP. *Pulmonary:* CTA, no wheeze/rhonchi/crackles. *Extremities:* no C/C/E

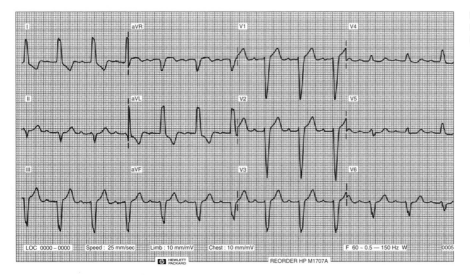

FIGURE 27 EKG with complete LBBB. (Image courtesy of S. Khayam-Bashi, MD.)

THOUGHT QUESTIONS
- What is the differential diagnosis of this patient's pain?
- Which diagnostic tests are indicated in this patient?
- What, if any, medicines do you need to prescribe this patient today?

Chest pain has a broad differential: respiratory disorders, GI (especially GERD), musculoskeletal, cardiac including aortic dissection and CAD), and psychiatric (anxiety disorder). The nature of this patient's chest pain points more to a cardiac source: occurs reproducibly with exercise, resolves with rest, not associated with eating.

This patient needs a functional study of her heart, as well as a cardiac risk assessment (including fasting lipid panel, basic metabolic panel, CBC, and diabetes screening—given her symptoms). Functional cardiac testing can be categorized by the stress given and the assessment tool used; see below.

There are also other combinations of the tests offered. In this patient, since she is able to exercise well but has LBBB on her EKG, as well as moderately convincing symptoms of angina, an exercise

TABLE 27. Cardiac Testing Options

TYPE OF TEST	STRESS	ASSESSMENT	EXCLUSIONS	ADVANTAGES	DISADVANTAGES
ETT: exercise treadmill test	Walking	EKG, BP, pulse, patient's symptoms	Poor exercise ability, pre-existing EKG abnormality, history of re-vascularization	Physiologic stress, least cost, less than one hour in length	Sensitivity and specificity lowest of all tests, especially in women and lower-risk patients; patient-effort dependent
Exercise sestamibi or exercise thallium	Walking	Primary: pre/post radionuclide perfusion imaging Secondary: EKG, BP, symptoms	Poor exercise ability	Physiologic stress; can locate area of heart with compromised perfusion	Increased cost; length of study at least four hours
Dipyridamole or adenosine sestamibi	Chemical vasodilators; unmask areas of coronary artery stenosis	Pre/post radionuclide perfusion imaging	Bronchospasm (from dipyridamole)	Can be performed on bed-bound hospitalized patients	Often two-day test; not a physiologic test, increased cost
Stress echocardiogram	Walking	Echocardiogram; assesses wall motion, overall ventricular function	Poor exercise ability	Physiologic stress, physiologic assessment; good prognostic indicator	Operator dependent; not offered at all institutions.
Dobutamine sestamibi/ dobutamine echo	Dobutamine—positive inotropic agent; induces ischemia	Pre/post radionuclide perfusion imaging or echocardiogram	Severe CHF	More physiologic stress than the chemical vasodilators	Not offered at all institutions, cost

sestamibi or exercise thallium would be indicated. An important point while you are waiting for her functional study and blood work is to educate the patient and her family regarding her health. She needs to be counseled on the signs and symptoms of coronary artery disease, and she should be encouraged not to smoke. You need to prescribe and educate her on the use of sublingual NTG PRN and aspirin qd. You can consider starting a low-dose beta blocker if you anticipate a wait for her study. Since this is her first visit to a doctor in the United States, most crucial is to establish a therapeutic alliance so that she will be comfortable returning to you and will follow up with her testing as indicated.

CASE CONTINUED

Your patient is scheduled for a functional study in one week. Her blood tests are: Total cholesterol: 260, LDL 170, TG 220, HDL 45. Fasting glucose 100; normal renal function, normal liver function tests. She returns to you in three days for a symptom check. Her blood pressure is 130/85. She has been feeling well, avoiding the hills that make her chest hurt, taking an aspirin. She has had no episodes of chest pain and has not needed NTG. You start her on pravastatin and arrange for phone follow-up with the patient and the cardiac testing lab after her test.

QUESTIONS

105. Which of the following is not a major risk factor for coronary artery disease?
    A. Smoking
    B. Diabetes mellitus
    C. Obesity
    D. Hypertension

106. If this patient proves to have coronary artery disease, what should be the goal of her lipid lowering therapy?
    A. LDL <100
    B. HDL >55
    C. Total cholesterol <200
    D. LDL <130

107. At the next visit, the patient's daughter brings in her own lab tests which were obtained at a free health fair two weeks prior. Her nonfasting results were: total cholesterol 240, HDL 60. You should:
    A. Prescribe her a cholesterol-reducing agent with laboratory follow-up in six weeks
    B. Give her a laboratory slip to have her fasting lipids and LFTs checked within a week, with close follow-up
    C. Prescribe her an aspirin and get an EKG
    D. Take a full medical history including diet and exercise, offer a nutrition referral, and schedule a follow-up appointment to discuss her health further

108. Which of the following side effects of aspirin would most affect how you would treat hypertension in this patient?
    A. GI bleed
    B. Angioedema
    C. Dyspepsia
    D. Tinnitus

ID/CC: A 58-year-old African-American man comes to his follow-up appointment complaining of difficulty breathing with increased cough.

HPI: SJ is a relatively new patient of yours with frequent visits. He has a history of "COPD/asthma" per the chart, with no intubations. He describes his baseline health as "OK—I can get around," but says that for the past two weeks he has been feeling increasingly short of breath and coughing more at night. His cough is productive of yellow sputum. No fever or chills.

PMHx: 1. HTN; no known end-organ damage. 2. BPH

Meds: 1. Albuterol MDI, two puffs q 6' PRN. 2. Atrovent MDI, two puffs qid. 3. HCTZ, 25 mg qd. 4. Prazosin, 4 mg qhs

All: NKDA   **Immunizations:** PPD negative last year, pneumovax two years prior

SHx: Lives with wife, teenage son. History of smoking 40 pack-year; quit one year ago. No alcohol or recreational drugs.

THOUGHT QUESTION
- What are other key points in the history; what aspects of the physical exam are important?

It is important to clarify this patient's pulmonary disease. Has he ever had pulmonary function tests? Does he have a baseline ABG? How often has he been using his inhalers? Is anyone else at home sick? Has he ever taken other medicines (including oral steroids) for his breathing? Does he use a peak flow meter to monitor his symptoms? Also, does he have any cardiac history? During the physical exam you should note his general appearance, his respiratory rate, temperature, and O_2 saturation. You should also check peak flow, and on his pulmonary exam look for accessory muscle use, listen carefully for a prolonged expiratory phase, and note any rhonchi or wheezes. Does he have other signs of chronic pulmonary disease like clubbing or hyperinflated chest?

Many patients with chronic lung disease will have some combination of chronic obstructive pulmonary disease and asthma, but pulmonary function testing will greatly assist with correct symptom and disease management.

Shaded=COPD

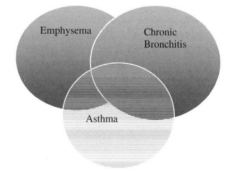

FIGURE 28 Venn diagram overlap.

CASE CONTINUED

VS: Temp 36.7°C. BP 135/85 HR 90 RR 20 O_2 Saturation 94% on RA PF: 250 (should be 500 based on height)

PE: *General:* slightly tired appearing gentleman, no respiratory distress. *Height:* 6'1". *Weight:* 160 pounds. *HEENT:* MMM, PERRL: no rhinorrhea, posterior O/P without lesions. *CV:* RR, rate at 90. No M/R/G. *Pulmonary:* I/E ratio 1:2; fair air movement, midexpiratory wheezes throughout. *Lung Fields:* No egophany. *Extremities:* no C/C/E.

You treat your patient with a nebulizer of albuterol and atrovent, after which his peak flow improves to 375 and his O_2 saturation goes to 96%. You arrange for quick follow-up and send him home with a short course of prednisone, in addition to his current MDIs (after administering an influenza vaccine).

QUESTIONS

109. In an isolated COPD exacerbation, short-term medical management includes all of the following except:
    A. Atrovent MDI round-the-clock
    B. Albuterol MDI as needed
    C. Treatment of bronchitis with antibiotics
    D. Corticosteroid MDI round-the-clock

110. All of the following regarding COPD are correct except:
    A. 50% of COPD cases can be linked to smoking
    B. COPD is airway obstruction caused by chronic bronchitis or emphysema
    C. COPD is the fourth leading cause of death in the United States
    D. Airway obstruction continues to worsen in patients who continue to smoke

111. All of the following regarding asthma is correct except:
    A. Asthma includes the triad of airway hyper-responsiveness, reversible bronchoconstriction, and inflammation
    B. Mild, intermittent asthma is characterized by symptoms more than weekly but less than daily with normal or near normal lung function
    C. Scheduled use of beta-2 agonists should be a part of treatment for mild intermittent asthma
    D. Treatment of asthma should be graded on the symptom severity

112. Pulmonary function tests would show the following:
    A. Decreased FEV1 for patients with COPD and asthma
    B. Increased DLCO if this patient has emphysema
    C. Decreased DLCO in a patient with an intracardiac shunt
    D. An increase in FEV1 of more than 5% and more than 75 ml in a patient with a "positive" response to a bronchodilator

ID/CC: A 42-year-old Chinese man comes to his annual clinic visit complaining of six weeks of cough.

HPI: LK had been feeling well until eight weeks prior when he had a "little cold." He had a fever for one day, then started feeling better. Since then, he has continued to have a cough sometimes productive of scant green mucus. He may have seen blood streaks in it once or twice. He denies any fevers, but has awakened sweaty a few times. His cough is there intermittently day and night, although it hasn't kept him from sleeping.

PMHx: 1. HTN. 2. DJD   **Meds:** HCTZ 25 mg qd

All: NKDA   **Immunizations:** PPD negative two years ago.

SHx: Emigrated from southern China five years ago; lives with wife, son, and daughter. Brother emigrated one and a half years ago and is living with them. Works in a food store.

Habits: Smoked 15 pack-year; quit 10 years ago.

VS: Temp 37.4°C BP 145/85 HR 80 RR 20 Sat 97% RA

PE: Thin Chinese man, NAD. *HEENT:* Normal nasal mucosa, no sinus TTP, TMs normal. *Neck:* No LAD. *CV:* RRR, no M/R/G. *Pulmonary:* Lungs CTA, no wheeze, rhonchi, or crackles. *Abdomen:* No hepatomegaly, nontender, nondistended. *Extremities:* No C/C/E.

THOUGHT QUESTIONS
- What is your differential diagnosis?
- What other studies are indicated today?

The differential diagnosis for chronic cough (cough lasting longer than three weeks) is broad, but fortunately can be narrowed by history and physical. The most common causes are asthma, postnasal drip, postinfectious, chronic bronchitis, and gastroesophageal reflux. More worrisome possible etiologies include bronchogenic carcinoma, tuberculosis, heart failure, and aortic aneurysm. Coughing due to an ACE-inhibitor causes an estimated 10% of ACE-taking patients to discontinue the medicine. Environmental irritants and smoking should also be investigated. In our patient above, certain elements stick out. His cough has lasted longer than a typical post-infectious cough. The fact that it is productive of green mucus raises the likelihood of ongoing infection, and the occasional blood streaks raise the risk of tuberculosis or carcinoma. Although he has a reassuringly normal physical exam, and his history is not that dramatic, he does need a chest x-ray and PPD placed today. (Even though he has a prior negative PPD, there has been a high-risk addition to his household.)

CASE CONTINUED

Your patient has a PPD placed and goes to get a chest x-ray. You get a report from the radiologist that the x-ray is normal. You inform your patient of this; you have a low suspicion of active TB. The patient agrees to continue without cough medicine until he comes back to get his PPD read. He returns in two days and his PPD measures 15 mm.

THOUGHT QUESTION
- What do you do now?

This patient is by definition a recent tuberculin converter (an increase in the size of the tuberculin reaction by at least 10 mm, and from less than 10 mm to 10 mm or more within a two-year period). Although his chest x-ray is normal, he is having possible tubercular symptoms and he must be treated as if he has active TB. Since you now have a moderately high suspicion of tuberculosis, he needs to be started on four-drug therapy (rifampin, PZA [pyrazinamide], ethambutol, and INH [isoniazid]) and have his sputum examined for evidence of tuberculosis. He is able to produce sputum independently, so after submitting three samples for acid fast bacteria smear and culture, he can go home with a TB mask. His family members need to be screened with a PPD.

CASE CONTINUED

Your patient has three AFB-negative smears and is continued on four-drug therapy. After eight weeks his cultures are negative for tuberculosis. His three-month follow-up CXR is still normal. He continues on INH and rifampin to complete a 16-week course.

QUESTIONS

113. The entire household has PPDs placed. The patient's daughter (age 18), who is asymptomatic, also has a positive PPD (14 mm). What intervention does she need?
    A. Sputum induction and four-drug therapy until cultures are negative
    B. Chest x-ray and six to nine months of INH
    C. An HIV test and 12 months of INH
    D. Chest x-ray and repeat PPD in six months

114. Which of the following patients taking INH do not require baseline and monthly liver function tests?
    A. Pregnant women
    B. HIV-infected patients
    C. Postpartum women of color
    D. Patients over the age of 35

115. Pyridoxine (vitamin B6) is routinely indicated as an adjunct to INH therapy in all of the following patients except:
    A. Children under age 15
    B. Patients with diabetes mellitus
    C. Alcoholics
    D. Patients with history of a seizure disorder

116. Patients with a history of BCG vaccine should have their tuberculosis screening altered in the following way:
    A. They should never have a PPD; instead they should have a screening CXR when symptomatic
    B. The BCG history should be ignored unless it was given within one year of the screening PPD
    C. The cutoff for positive PPD is greater than 15 mm in a patient with prior BCG
    D. If the BCG was given more than 10 years prior, they can be screened as normal

CASE 30 / DYSPNEA ON EXERTION

ID/CC: LF is a 36-year-old Samoan female who presents to your clinic as a new patient, brought in by her husband who is also your patient.

HPI: LF recently moved to the United States from American Samoa three months ago. She migrated to the U.S. to be reunited with her husband, an American citizen, and her four children who had moved earlier. She has no complaints at this time, and merely wants a checkup. She is happy to be reunited with her husband and children, and says she wants to have another child.

PMHx: Notes that she had rheumatic fever as a child, but denies any other illnesses

Meds: None   **All:** NKDA   **FHx:** HTN—both parents

SHx: Lives with husband, their four children (ages 15, 13, 12, and 9), and her in-laws (mother-in-law, father-in-law, sister-in-law), unemployed at this time, finished high school in American Samoa, worked as a housekeeper in Samoa.

ROS: LF has no spontaneous complaints, but further questioning reveals increasing dyspnea on exertion, malaise, and fatigue, which LF attributes to jet lag and the adjustment to a new country. No CP, no palpitations, no abdominal complaints, no fever, chills, night sweats, or weight loss. No paroxysmal nocturnal dyspnea, no orthopnea.

VS: Afebrile   BP 120/70   HR 64   RR 18   100% RA

PE: *Gen:* No respiratory distress. *Skin:* no rashes, no jaundice. *HEENT:* no JVD. *CV:* irregularly irregular rhythm at 96, IV/VI holosystolic murmur at the apex. *Chest:* CTA bilaterally, no rales. *Abdomen:* benign. *Extremities:* radial pulses 2+ at 64; no cyanosis/clubbing/edema. *Neuro:* nonfocal

---

THOUGHT QUESTIONS
- What is the cause of the murmur?
- What is the cause of LF's dyspnea on exertion?

The murmur is secondary to LF's childhood rheumatic fever, and probable rheumatic carditis at the time. Rheumatic fever can cause scarring of the heart valves, most commonly mitral and tricuspid. She has the classic apical holosystolic murmur of mitral regurgitation. Her dyspnea on exertion is caused by mild congestive heart failure with volume overload into the pulmonary vasculature, and the inability of her heart to maintain cardiac output secondary to valvular dysfunction.

CASE CONTINUED

Because of her "pulse deficit" (the difference between the rates of the apical and peripheral pulses), and her irregularly irregular rhythm, an EKG is obtained in the office.

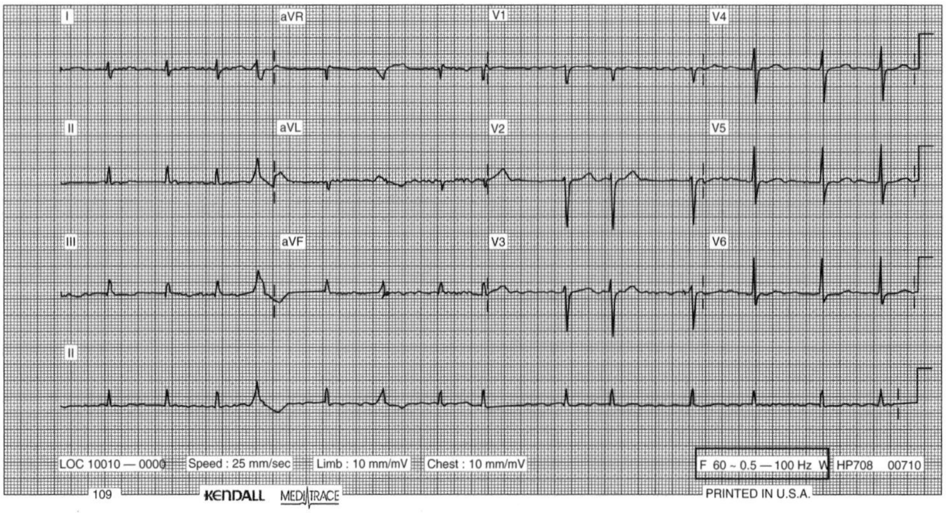

FIGURE 30 EKG of atrial fibrillation.

THOUGHT QUESTIONS

- What does the EKG show?
- How would you manage this patient?

The EKG shows an irregularly irregular rhythm without distinct P waves; an EKG characteristic of atrial fibrillation. The patient is in chronic atrial fibrillation due to mitral valve dysfunction. Management of chronic atrial fibrillation focuses on two areas: 1) controlling symptoms from the arrhythmia (rate control), and 2) decreasing the risk for thromboembolism (anticoagulation). Rate control can be achieved with a beta blocker, a calcium-channel blocker, or digoxin. Anticoagulation in this young patient should be maintained with warfarin. Warfarin is more effective than aspirin in decreasing thromboembolic events, but does have an increased risk for bleeding, including hemorrhagic strokes. If warfarin is prescribed, the family physician must discuss issues of family planning and contraception, as warfarin is highly teratogenic.

QUESTIONS

117. Which of the following statements regarding digoxin is false?
    A. Digoxin toxicity includes visual changes, gastrointestinal effects, and alterations in the serum potassium level
    B. Digoxin administration to patients with atrial fibrillation requires frequent monitoring of therapeutic serum levels
    C. EKG changes with digoxin toxicity include ventricular tachycardia, ventricular fibrillation, and junctional tachyarrhythmias
    D. Digoxin is derived from the foxglove plant

118. Which clinical scenario does not indicate an early electrical cardioversion?
    A. A 50-year-old female with no significant past medical history presents to the ED with a one-day history of acute onset palpitations, and atrial fibrillation on EKG
    B. A 63-year-old male with past medical history significant for coronary artery disease presents to the ED with anginal chest pain, and new atrial fibrillation on EKG compared with a day-old EKG demonstrating normal sinus rhythm
    C. A 69-year-old male in atrial fibrillation with a ventricular response rate of 140, a blood pressure of 80/40, who presents feeling dizzy and weak, with poor peripheral pulses on exam
    D. A 77-year-old female with a two-week history of atrial fibrillation, on oral anticoagulation for one week, without evidence of atrial thrombus on echocardiogram, who is rate-controlled with metoprolol

119. Which valve is most commonly affected in rheumatic heart disease?
    A. Aortic valve
    B. Pulmonic valve
    C. Mitral valve
    D. Tricuspid valve

120. Which of the following statements regarding atrial fibrillation is false?
    A. Atrial fibrillation is the most common arrhythmia
    B. Atrial fibrillation is a major risk factor for stroke
    C. Asthmatic patients taking theophylline or beta-agonists, without any underlying cardiac disease, may experience transient episodes of atrial fibrillation
    D. The atrial rate in atrial fibrillation is approximately 200 beats/minute

CASE 31 / SMOKER WITH URI

ID/CC: A 45-year-old patient comes in for a URI. You glance through his chart and see that he smokes.

HPI: The patient has had typical URI symptoms for two days, and is complaining of a cough and sore throat. His cough is productive of whitish sputum and he has burning chest pain when he coughs. He denies chest pain with walking up hills or stairs. He complains of rhinorrhea and occasional ear pain. He feels achy and may have had a low-grade temperature last night.

He has smoked one pack per day for 20 years and has never before tried to quit although his wife and kids have been asking him to. He states that his doctors have never brought up quitting in the past. He admits that he does not have regular medical care but just uses the urgent care whenever necessary. He had bronchitis twice last winter and does not want to get that sick again. He was hoping for some early antibiotics this time "to nip it in the bud." He is tired and stressed out and feels that another bout of bronchitis would push him over the edge.

PMHx: Hypertension, chronic hepatitis C

PSHx: Knee surgery 10 years ago, ex-lap for GSW 20 years ago

Meds: Atenolol 50 mg per day, ASA 81 mg per day **All:** NKDA

SHx: One beer per day, one pack per day tobacco, occasional marijuana, history of heroin use 20 years ago

Married with two children

THOUGHT QUESTION

- What is the most important question to ask during the visit?

70% of smokers see doctors regularly, and multiple studies show that quit rates increase with physician involvement and simple questioning about smoking cessation.

The National Cancer Institute recommends the program of "4 As" at each visit with a smoker:

—Ask about smoking
—Advise about smoking cessation
—Assist with smoking cessation
—Arrange for follow-up

Smoking causes 6–15% of *all* health care costs. 38% of all cancer deaths in men and 23% of all cancer deaths in women are related to cigarettes. Smoking accounts for 80–85% of cases of COPD, and is related to a large proportion of heart disease.

VS: Temp 99°F BP 158/90 HR 65 RR 20 Sat 95% RA

PE: Very anxious thin man, jittery and stuttering a bit. *Weight:* 140. *Height:* 5'11'. *OP:* Erythematous without exudate, TM clear bilaterally, neck supple without LAD. *Lungs:* Coarse with occasional wheezes and crackles bilaterally, CV RRR without murmur. *Abdomen:* Soft, nontender, no HSM, no Murphy's. *Extremities:* No edema.

THOUGHT QUESTION

• The patient is pressuring you for a prescription. How likely is he to get one?

Antibiotic overuse and abuse is an increasingly disturbing problem in medicine and in public health and is the main cause of the spread of antibiotic-resistant bacteria. The most concerning problem and the easiest to target is the overuse of antibiotics for URIs, colds, bronchitis, otitis, and pharyngitis. In most cases, these infections are of viral etiology and are self-limited. Interestingly, recent studies found that residents are less likely to prescribe antibiotics for colds, URIs, and bronchitis than are attending physicians.

Factors implicated in unnecessary drug usage include time pressures, patient pressure and expectations, diagnostic uncertainty, patient inability to comply with follow-up, misinformation on the diagnosis of viral versus bacterial infections of the head and neck, free antibiotic samples from drug representatives, and advertising aimed directly at patients.

Physicians seem to equate patient satisfaction with an antibiotic prescription; however, recent studies suggest that patient satisfaction correlates more closely with a careful explanation of the symptoms, time with the patient, and time to answer the patient's questions and concerns.

QUESTIONS

121. The patient is sheepish about his smoking, and states that he wants to quit but is scared of the withdrawal symptoms, which include all of the following EXCEPT:
    A. Bradycardia
    B. Impaired concentration
    C. Weight loss
    D. Depression

122. You reassure the patient that there are both pharmacologic and behavioral approaches to aid in smoking cessation, including:
    A. Psychotherapy
    B. Nicotine candy cigarettes
    C. Buproprion
    D. Antabuse

123. Although it is only a 15-minute visit, after speaking with the patient about smoking cessation, you suspect that he is also depressed. Criteria for a diagnosis of major depression include all of the following EXCEPT:
    A. Increased libido
    B. Weight gain
    C. Insomnia
    D. Feelings of worthlessness

124. You give the patient acetaminophen and a decongestant for his cold, and set a smoking quit date in one week. You start him on nicotine patches and buproprion, and tell him that if his depression doesn't respond appropriately to buproprion, the drug class of choice for depression with anxiety is considered to be:
    A. Benzodiazepines
    B. SSRIs (serotonin selective reuptake inhibitors)
    C. TCAs (tricyclic antidepressants)
    D. St. John's wort (*hypericum*)

ID/CC: A 56-year-old Chinese woman comes to her regularly scheduled healthcare maintenance appointment complaining of two weeks of a gradually increasing swollen right leg.

HPI: TC is a patient well-known to you; she is very stoic and rarely complains. She describes for the past two weeks noticing that her right sock was tight, then seeing redness and swelling in her right shin and calf. It bothers her some, mostly with an achy feeling. She denies shortness of breath, chest pain, change in exercise tolerance, and recent travel; no trauma or fever or chills, no nausea or vomiting; no weight loss.

PMHx: 1. HTN diagnosed six months ago. 2. eczema.   **PSHx:** None

Meds: 1. Premarin 0.625 mg/Provera 2.5 mg qd. 2. HCTZ 25 mg qd. 3. triamcinolone cream. Healthcare maintenance: UTD

All: NKDA   **FHx:** No clotting disorders.

SHx: Works as an aide in a preschool; lives with husband and 20-year-old son. No tobacco, no alcohol, no recreational drugs. Emigrated from China nine years ago.

VS: BP 140/85 HR 75 RR 16 Sat 99% RA

PE: *Gen:* no distress, walking without difficulty. *CV:* RRR, no M/R/G. *Pulmonary:* CTA. *Extremities:* RLE with 1+ pitting edema and erythema to mid-calf; mildly TTP. No hyperpigmentation. No cords palpable; negative Homan sign. DP/PT pulses 2+. LLE no C/C/E. Circumference of calf 10 cm below tibial tubercle: right: 35 cm; left: 30 cm.

THOUGHT QUESTIONS

- What is the differential diagnosis for TC's problem?
- What additional workup does she need?
- What factors in her history may help you?

Bilateral lower extremity swelling, a common problem, generates a broad differential diagnosis, including CHF, hypoalbuminemia (from liver or kidney disease), venous stasis, lymphedema, medicine side effect (for example, calcium channel blockers and alpha-methyldopa), and pulmonary hypertension. Unilateral presentation could be one of the above presenting in an atypical fashion, but should also raise the question of venous thromboembolism. Risk factors for venous thromboembolism include immobility, surgery (especially orthopedic), smoking, pregnancy, underlying malignancy, old age, hormonal supplementation, and clotting disorders. Our patient above has a known risk factor of hormone replacement therapy (which increases the risk of thromboembolism in a postmenopausal woman by three to four times).

History and physical exam for deep venous thromboembolism are notoriously poor: 50–75% of patients who present with clinically suspected DVT have nonthrombotic causes of leg pain. However, morbidity and mortality of untreated DVT are high, and therefore a more definitive study is indicated. Doppler-flow ultrasonography with a vein compression test is the best first-line study. For venous thromboembolism above the knee, its sensitivity and specificity are above 97%. For thromboembolism below the knee, it is much less accurate.

CASE CONTINUED

TC gets an ultrasound study across town at the hospital and returns to wait. You receive the report that she has reduced blood flow with a clot in her popliteal vein that extends superiorly for approximately 10 cm.

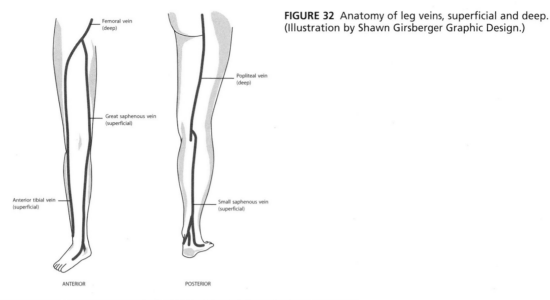

FIGURE 32 Anatomy of leg veins, superficial and deep. (Illustration by Shawn Girsberger Graphic Design.)

Femoral vein (deep)

Popliteal vein (deep)

Great saphenous vein (superficial)

Anterior tibial vein (superficial)

Small saphenous vein (superficial)

ANTERIOR   POSTERIOR

THOUGHT QUESTIONS

• What do you tell your patient now?
• What are options for treatment?
• What further workup and testing are indicated?

TC does have a proximal deep venous thrombosis, which untreated would have a very high morbidity and mortality. (Although impossible to study now, retrospective analyses indicate that between 15% and 30% of patients with untreated DVT may die from fatal pulmonary embolism.) This patient has two options for treatment: hospitalization with intravenous unfractionated heparin followed by Coumadin, or outpatient treatment with subcutaneous low-molecular-weight heparin (LMWH) with either transition to coumadin or continued LMWH. The workup for cause of first-time thrombosis should be tailored for each patient. This patient should be counseled regarding the risks and benefits of continuing her HRT. In the patient with no known risk factors, it is worthwhile to test for factor V Leiden and prothrombin mutations, as this will affect treatment length and family counseling. Although patients with cancer do have a higher risk of DVT, it is not necessary to do additional cancer testing in a patient with a clot who has received all usual screening tests.

QUESTIONS

125. This patient should be anticoagulated for:
    A. One month
    B. Two months
    C. Three to six months
    D. Life

126. The goal INR for treatment of DVT with Coumadin is:
    A. 1.5–2.0
    B. 2–3
    C. 3–4
    D. 4–4.5

127. A different patient comes to your office with a similar history and physical, but on ultrasound has a "technically limited study" that does not reveal any abnormalities. You should:
    A. Counsel her extensively and repeat the ultrasound study in one week
    B. Schedule her for a venogram as soon as possible, but definitely within three days
    C. Order lab tests including fibrin, fibrinogen, and D-dimers
    D. Reassure her and ask her to call for an appointment if her leg isn't better in two to three months

128. Low-molecular-weight heparin (LMWH) is contraindicated in all of the following scenarios except:
    A. Renal failure
    B. Weight greater than 100 kg
    C. Retroperitoneal bleed
    D. Diabetes

ID/CC: AT is a 67-year-old African-American female who presents to her PMD complaining of "tingling feet."

HPI: AT had been otherwise well until about four months ago when she started noticing a tingling sensation in her feet. She describes the sensation as if her feet had "fallen asleep," which used to happen when she sat for prolonged periods of time at her desk years ago. The sensation has been more constant in the recent months, and now she even feels it at night. She doesn't know what is causing the symptom, otherwise feels well, and denies any recent illnesses.

PMHx: Vitiligo for 20 years

Graves disease status post I^{131} ablation 35 years ago, now hypothyroid

Meds: Levothyroxine 0.125 mcg daily, acetaminophen as needed

All: Ibuprofen causes hives   **FHx:** Mother DM 2 – alive at 88 years old; did not know her father

SHx: Lives with her husband, retired paralegal, five children, eight grandchildren

Habits: No tobacco, no drugs, occasional social alcohol

ROS: Upon further questioning, the patient reveals that she has been feeling more fatigued recently, with some forgetfulness, dizziness, with a few intermittent bouts of diarrhea in the past month with a five-pound weight loss. She denies any fever, chills, night sweats, melena, bright red blood per rectum, chest pain, shortness of breath.

VS: Afebrile BP 124/72 HR 110 RR 18 O_2 Saturation 100% on RA

PE: *Gen:* no acute distress. *Skin:* multiple depigmented areas over face, trunk, extremities. *HEENT:* no scleral icterus, smooth tongue. *Neck:* no masses. *CV:* tachycardic with a II/VI systolic ejection murmur over upper left sternal border. *Chest:* CTA bilaterally. *Abdomen:* benign. *Extremities:* no cyanosis/clubbing/edema. *Neuro:* CN II-XII intact, motor exam reveals 5/5 strength in upper and lower extremities bilaterally, decreased position sensation of toes bilaterally, decreased vibratory sensation to the ankles bilaterally, cerebellar testing of finger-to-nose is intact, positive Romberg test. *Reflexes:* 2+ biceps/triceps/brachioradialis bilaterally, 1+ patellar/ankle bilaterally, positive Babinski bilaterally

Laboratory tests are ordered and the results return in one week at the patient's follow-up visit significant for: Hgb 9.4 g/dL (Nl 12–16), Hct 28% (Nl 37–48), MCV 112 fL (Nl 80–100), peripheral smear: 1+ anisocytosis, 2+ macroovalocytes

---

THOUGHT QUESTIONS

- What is the differential for macrocytic anemia?
- What is the most likely diagnosis?

The differential diagnosis for macrocytic anemia is acute hemorrhage or hemolysis (reticulocytosis), vitamin B12 deficiency (malabsorption, disorders of the terminal ileum, intestinal flora competition, drugs), folic acid deficiency (increased requirements, malabsorption, impaired metabolism), or drugs that impair DNA metabolism. Given the neurologic findings, the patient has a vitamin B12 deficiency, with the complication of subacute combined degeneration of the cord. This is an upper motor neuron deficit caused by posterior column involvement with peripheral nerve and spinal neuron demyelination causing a myelopathy, mental changes, and peripheral neuropathy.

CASE CONTINUED

Additional laboratory data reveals: Serum vitamin B12 level: 88 pg/mL (decreased). RBC-folate level: 15 mg/mL (normal). Decreased reticulocyte count

A Schilling test is performed, showing an abnormal first stage, and a normal second stage, indicating pernicious anemia with an intrinsic factor deficiency.

THOUGHT QUESTION

• Discuss the Schilling test.

The Schilling test evaluates the etiology of vitamin B12 deficiency. It is performed in two stages. In the first stage, a patient is given PO radioactive cobalamin, and then administered an unlabeled intramuscular injection of cobalamin. A 24-hour urine collection reveals the proportion of radioactive cobalamin excreted. This first stage should always be abnormal, since cobalamin deficiency is almost always due to malabsorption. In the second stage, the patient is given radioactive cobalamin bound to intrinsic factor. If the absorption is normal, the patient has pernicious anemia or other intrinsic factor deficiency. If the absorption is still abnormal, the patient has either bacterial overgrowth competing for the vitamin or some type of ileal disease.

QUESTIONS

129. The appropriate treatment for pernicious anemia is:
    A. Oral administration of folic acid
    B. Intramuscular administration of intrinsic factor
    C. Oral administration of vitamin B12
    D. Intramuscular administration of vitamin B12

130. Which of the following is not a cause of vitamin B12 deficiency?
    A. Infestation by *Diphyllobothrium latum*
    B. Strict vegetarianism
    C. Gastrectomy
    D. Zidovudine administration

131. Which of the following can be seen on the peripheral smear of a patient with pernicious anemia?
    A. Hypersegmented neutrophils
    B. Ringed sideroblasts
    C. Sickle-shaped red blood cells
    D. Band neutrophils with Dohle bodies

132. Clinical signs and symptoms of megaloblastic anemia caused by folic acid deficiency would not include:
    A. Pallor and tachycardia
    B. Decreased vibratory sensation
    C. Cheilosis and glossitis
    D. Malnourished appearance

CASE 34 / ANKLE SWELLING

ID/CC: TH is a 70-year-old African-American male who presents to his regular physician complaining of "ankle swelling that comes and goes" for the past five months.

HPI: TH has noticed ankle swelling since his last visit six months ago. He has no pain in his joints, and can't recall any particular trauma to his legs. No redness, warmth, or other affected joints. The swelling lasts for about three to five days at a time, occurring randomly about seven times in the previous five months. The patient discovered that the swelling goes away when he elevates his legs and limits salty foods. The patient is currently asymptomatic.

PMHx: CAD with anterolateral MI five years ago, s/p PTCA with stent placement in proximal RCA for 70% occlusion, HTN, hypercholesterolemia, cataracts

ROS: No fever, chills, night sweats, heat or cold intolerance, no chest pain, + fatigue, + dyspnea on exertion to two blocks, + paroxysmal nocturnal dyspnea, + two pillow orthopnea, + nocturia

Meds: ASA 325 mg daily, Atenolol 100 mg daily, Simvastatin 40 mg once at bedtime, Benazepril 40 mg daily

All: Penicillin causes anaphylaxis   **FHx:** Father died of MI at 59 years old, son has HTN

SHx: Lives with wife, son, and daughter-in-law, retired chef

Habits: 60 pack per year tobacco history, two to three glasses of wine per week

VS: Afebrile BP 138/88 HR 60 RR 18 O_2 Saturation 100% on RA

PE: *Gen:* no acute distress, well-developed/well-nourished. *HEENT:* within normal limits. *Neck:* no JVD. *CV:* RRR no murmurs/gallops/rubs, + faint S4. *Chest:* CTA bilaterally. *Abdomen:* protuberant, BS+, soft, nontender, no organomegaly. *Extremities:* no edema, dorsalis pedis and posterior tibialis pulses 2+ bilaterally

---

THOUGHT QUESTION

- Explain the patient's symptomatology. What diagnostic study would you order?

Given the patient's medical history of myocardial infarction and hypertension, the most likely cause of his constellation of symptoms is congestive heart failure. The patient's symptoms are consistent with total volume overload into the pulmonary vasculature ("congestion"), as well as decreased cardiac output ("failure"), secondary to left ventricular dysfunction. Decreased cardiac output leads to reflexive physiologic neurohumoral changes: sodium retention, increased peripheral resistance, and increased catecholamine release, all due to what the kidneys sense as "low" intravascular volume. The neurohumoral changes ultimately result in water retention and total volume overload from sodium retention, arrhythmias from catecholamine stimulation, and further impedance to cardiac output from increased peripheral resistance.

Diagnosis of CHF rests upon signs and symptoms and evaluation of cardiac function via echocardiography or radionuclide angiography. An echocardiogram is the most useful study because it will document size and function of atria and ventricles, estimate ejection fraction, and reveal wall motion abnormalities in contrast to dilated cardiomyopathy; it can also distinguish between systolic and diastolic dysfunction. Radionuclide angiography is more invasive, but would be more useful when an echocardiogram is suboptimal.

CASE CONTINUED

A transthoracic echocardiogram reveals:

1. segmental left ventricular and septal wall motion abnormalities
2. moderate concentric left ventricular hypertrophy .
3. left ventricular dysfunction with an estimated ejection fraction of 35%
4. mild relaxation abnormality
5. normal valves

THOUGHT QUESTIONS
- What kind of heart failure does this patient have?
- What is the difference between systolic and diastolic dysfunction?

This patient has features of both systolic and diastolic failure or dysfunction. His systolic dysfunction (primarily ventricular "pump" failure) is manifested as left ventricular failure, seen on echocardiogram as a low EF and segmental wall motion abnormalities. He also has a component of diastolic dysfunction, seen as a relaxation abnormality (a "stiff" ventricle that cannot relax, with resultant increased diastolic pressures transmitted into the pulmonary vasculature). Patients may experience the same symptoms for both types of dysfunction (dyspnea, orthopnea, fatigue). Treatments for systolic and diastolic dysfunction differ, however, and it is important to establish the type of CHF.

TABLE 34. Treatment of Systolic Dysfunction	
GOAL OF TREATMENT	**MEDICATION**
Symptom control	Loop diuretics
Afterload reduction	ACE inhibitors
	Hydralazine with nitrates
Neurohumoral blockade	Beta-blockers
	Potassium-sparing diuretics
Increased Inotropy	Digoxin

Treatment of Diastolic Dysfunction – theoretical goal of increasing cardiac filling time (via diastole) to improve cardiac output, via beta blockers or calcium-channel blockers.

QUESTIONS

133. Which of the following statements is false?
    A. CHF is the largest single medical diagnosis for hospital admissions in the United States.
    B. Morbidity and mortality from CHF in African-Americans are equivalent to that of Caucasian-Americans
    C. CHF morbidity and mortality have increased secondary to a decline in coronary artery disease and hypertension mortality
    D. Coronary artery disease is the most common cause of CHF in developed countries

134. Which of the following heart sounds is a sign of an acute exacerbation of congestive heart failure?
    A. Split S1
    B. Split S2
    C. S3
    D. S4

135. Which of the therapeutic modalities is not used to treat systolic dysfunction CHF?
    A. Loop diuretics
    B. Angiotensin converting enzyme inhibitors
    C. Potassium-sparing diuretics
    D. Angiotensin receptor blockers

136. Which of the following classes of medications has not shown a mortality benefit in CHF?
    A. ACE inhibitors
    B. Beta blockers
    C. Potassium-sparing diuretics
    D. Loop diuretics

ID/CC: JR is a 58-year-old Caucasian male who presents to his regularly scheduled clinic appointment complaining of three days of severe right knee pain.

HPI: The patient is a heavy-set, stoic gentleman who reports that he began having right knee pain and swelling since Sunday night (three days ago). He has never experienced this pain before, but thought that his symptoms might be due to tripping and landing on his knees the day before. It hurts to bend his knee and walking is difficult. There has been no improvement despite using ibuprofen and icing his knee. He also notes that he felt "a little warm," and had a mild cough, sore throat, and irritated, watery eyes since last week.

PMHx: Hyperlipidemia, hypertension, DM 2, osteoarthritis, seasonal allergies   **PSHx:** None

Meds: Ibuprofen as needed, pravastatin 20 mg once at bedtime, hydrochlorothiazide 25 mg once a day, ASA 81 mg daily, metformin 500 mg three times a day

All: NKDA   **ROS:** Above   **FHx:** Father MI 67 years old, sister DM 2

SHx: Mechanic, lives with wife, smokes one pack per day tobacco, alcohol every weekend with his friends

VS: Temp 38.2°C BP 164/92 HR 88 RR 16

PE: Obese male, limping into office, right knee erythematous, swollen, warm, severe tenderness to palpation, otherwise normal exam

---

THOUGHT QUESTION

- What is included in the differential diagnosis? What laboratory test would be most useful in determining the cause of knee pain and swelling?

The differential diagnosis for monoarticular arthritis is large; more likely causes in this febrile patient with an acute onset, lower extremity monoarticular arthritis include gout, pseudogout, septic arthritis, and Reiter's syndrome. Knee inflammation eliminates osteoarthritis as the primary cause. Gout, pseudogout, septic arthritis, and Reiter's syndrome are all inflammatory arthritides. Gout is associated with obesity, hypertension, hyperlipidemia, and DM, usually affecting middle-aged or elderly men; it can present in any joint, but usually affects the first metatarsalphalangeal joint (podagra) or knees in first presentation. Pseudogout (calcium pyrophosphate dihydrate crystals) can develop due to severe osteoarthritis, but can also be a hereditary disease. Septic arthritis is possible in the patient with DM; gram-negative organisms would be most common. Reiter's syndrome is more likely if the patient presents with the triad of arthritis, conjunctivitis, and urethritis. He has irritated, watery eyes, but does not exhibit conjunctivitis.

An arthrocentesis to analyze the synovial fluid is necessary. The synovial fluid should be sent for cell count, glucose, stat Gram stain, bacterial culture, and inspection for crystals under polarized microscopy.

Labs: 30 cc cloudy fluid aspirated, 50,000 WBCs – 78% neutrophils, 2000 RBCs, glucose WNL, positive for needle-shaped negatively birefringent crystals on polarized microscopy, no organisms seen on Gram stain, culture pending

---

THOUGHT QUESTIONS

• What is the diagnosis?

• What are key characteristics you would have expected for the other diagnoses?

This patient has gout, proven by the needle-shaped negatively birefringent crystals on polarized microscopy, in conjunction with his clinical presentation. The urate crystals may be intracellular and extracellular within the synovial fluid. An elevated white cell count between 10,000 and 60,000 is characteristic, with a predominance of neutrophils.

Evidence of other diagnoses would be:

Pseudogout – weakly positively birefringent rhomboid-shaped crystals under polarized microscopy, either intracellular or extracellular. Fluid leukocytosis would be less—between 10,000 and 20,000 is characteristic, again predominantly neutrophils.

Septic arthritis – leukocytosis averaging 50,000 with neutrophil predominance. Gram stain may reveal organisms, more commonly in nongonococcal arthritis. Decreased synovial fluid glucose.

Reiter's syndrome – non-specific leukocytosis, no other special characteristics. Serum HLA-B27 positive in 80% of patients.

QUESTIONS

137. Which of the following medications listed below should be used for this patient's acute gout attack?
    A. Allopurinol
    B. Probenecid
    C. Aspirin
    D. Colchicine

138. Which of the following diagnostic studies would not be useful in determining pharmaceutical treatment in a patient with tophaceous gout:
    A. Arthrocentesis during an attack
    B. Serum uric acid value
    C. 24-hour urine collection
    D. Creatinine clearance

139. Which of the following circumstances would not have contributed to this patient's gout?
    A. Falling on his knees one day prior to onset
    B. Drinking alcohol during the weekend with his friends
    C. Taking hydrochlorothiazide for hypertension
    D. Taking aspirin for primary prevention of cardiovascular disease
    E. Taking ibuprofen for symptomatic relief of fever

140. In 10 years this patient would not exhibit which of the following clinical and diagnostic features?
    A. Nodules on the pinna of the ears
    B. Radiography of the knee revealing bony erosion
    C. Abdominal radiography revealing nephrolithiasis
    D. Chronic inflammation of involved joints

ID/CC: OA is a 53-year-old woman complaining of right knee pain.

HPI: The patient has had knee pain on and off for the past five years. "In fact, now that you are asking," she interjects, "my fingers bother me in the mornings, and my hips can ache something terrible on rainy days. Can you give me a pill and cure it please?" The patient describes the pain as deep and aching, and worse when she has been walking a lot or going up and down stairs. Occasionally she even feels like her knee will give out on her.

PMHx: CAD; inferior wall MI two years ago, hyperlipidemia, obesity, PUD

PSHx: Herniorrhaphy 30 years ago, Lap cholecystectomy 10 years ago

Meds: Pravastatin 20 mg qd, metoprolol 50 mg qd, ASA 325 mg qd, Vit E 400 IU qd, fosinopril 20 mg qd, lansoprazole 30 mg qd

All: NKDA

THOUGHT QUESTION
• Joint pain and stiffness suggest what differential diagnosis?

All rheumatic diseases share the symptoms of pain and joint stiffness, and can be broadly subdivided into: osteoarthritis, inflammatory arthritis (rheumatoid arthritis, ankylosing spondylitis, gout, pseudogout, etc.), diffuse connective tissue disease (SLE, etc.), and musculoskeletal syndromes (bursitis, tendonitis, fibromyalgia, etc.).

VS: Temp 98°F BP 134/82 HR 70 RR 12

PE: Well-nourished obese woman, appears well. Weight 210 Height 5'5". Right knee moderately tender to palpation at joint line, crepitus with flexion and slightly decreased ROM, no erythema or effusion, no instability. Left knee WNL. Moderate enlargement of PIP and DIP joints with good ROM, nontender. Rest of PE WNL.

THOUGHT QUESTION
• What are risk factors for knee osteoarthritis?

Risk factors include:

- female gender (older than 50 years 1.7 times higher risk than men)
- postmenopausal/estrogen deficiency?
- obesity: with each 10 pound weight gain risk increases 40%, with each 10 pound weight loss risk decreases 40%
- quadricep weakness
- joint laxity with age-associated increase in varus-valgus laxity
- genetic
- heavy physical activity

THOUGHT QUESTION
- How do nutritional supplements help treat osteoarthritis these days?

Glucosamine and chondroitin have been used in Europe for many years to help alleviate the symptoms of arthritis. Glucosamine is an aminomonosaccharide, which is a constituent of the glycoprotein, proteoglycans, glycosaminoglycans, and other building blocks of connective tissue, including articular cartilage. In vitro studies show that glucosamine is incorporated into human chondrocytes and also stimulates proteoglycan synthesis; it is also a mild anti-inflammatory. Trials have shown improved symptoms, range of motion, swelling, and tenderness to palpation with glucosamine supplementation. In trials comparing glucosamine with ibuprofen or acetaminophen, it appears to be equal or slightly better than these medications, has far fewer side effects, and fewer patients on glucosamine dropped out of the studies. Scanning electron micrographs of cartilage suggest that glucosamine not only treats symptoms but also helps with *rebuilding* of cartilage.

Chondroitin is a component of the glycosaminoglycans that maintain viscosity in joints. It also stimulates cartilage repair and inhibits the enzyme that degrades cartilage. Like glucosamine, it has anti-inflammatory properties. It is a much larger molecule than glucosamine and therefore is poorly absorbed: 10% of a dose of chondroitin is absorbed vs. more than 90% of glucosamine. Far fewer studies have assessed the effects of chondroitin in vivo, and it is often paired with glucosamine, but it appears to help decrease symptoms and possibly help with cartilage repair.

Most physicians prescribe both together, and many OTC brands of the combination are available in pharmacies and supermarkets.

QUESTIONS

141. Which of the following is NOT typical of osteoarthritis?
    A. Joint stiffness on awakening that lasts for 20 to 30 minutes
    B. Osteophytes
    C. Bone cysts
    D. Joint effusions and localized warmth

142. Which joints are most commonly affected with osteoarthritis?
    A. Spine
    B. Toes
    C. Elbows
    D. Shoulders

143. The gold standard diagnostic test for osteoarthritis is:
    A. X-ray
    B. MRI
    C. Joint aspiration
    D. There isn't one

144. The keystone of therapy for osteoarthritis is
    A. Joint replacement
    B. Nonpharmacologic (exercise, joint protection, weight loss, thermal rx, etc.)
    C. Anti-inflammatory medications
    D. Acetaminophen

ID/CC: AH is a 32-year-old female who presents to the acute care clinic complaining that "I have a urine infection and I need a prescription for antibiotics."

HPI: The patient reports that she is having a UTI – she has had them in the past, and the symptoms now are the same as before. She has urinary frequency, mild dysuria, slight low back and abdominal pain, a low-grade fever, and mild nausea, but no vomiting. No past hospitalizations for her infections. The symptoms began at work today, but she could not leave work in time to visit her regular physician. There have been four episodes like this in the past, all of which responded well to pills; the last episode occurred two months ago. She uses condoms with every intercourse, and denies any STDs.

PMHx: UTIs in the past   **PSHx:** Appendectomy age 11   **Meds:** Acetaminophen

All: NKDA   **FHx:** Noncontributory   **SHx:** Receptionist   **ROS:** No diarrhea, no vaginal discharge

VS: Temp 38.1°C BP 128/70 HR 72 RR 16

PE: Mild discomfort with exam, but otherwise nontoxic appearance. *Abdomen:* BS present, mild suprapubic tenderness, no peritoneal signs. *Back:* mild costovertebral angle tenderness present on the left. *Udip:* pH 8, + RBCs, + leukocytes, + esterase, + protein, otherwise negative. *Stat Gram stain:* swarming short gram-negative rods

---

THOUGHT QUESTIONS

- What is the diagnosis?
- What would your management be at this point?

The patient has pyelonephritis, likely caused by *Proteus* species (characteristic Gram stain of swarming short gram-negative rods). She is nontoxic, so could be managed as an outpatient with close follow-up, especially with her history of responding well to oral antibiotics. If treated as an outpatient with close follow-up, the urine should be sent for culture and sensitivities, and as in this patient, a Gram stain and formal urinalysis should be obtained. The Gram stain is helpful in identifying a preliminary organism (e.g., *E. coli* is described as thick/fat gram-negative rods) and could narrow the spectrum of antibiotics prescribed. Communication with her PMD to ensure an outpatient workup for recurrent urinary tract infections is ideal. The patient should receive broad-spectrum antibiotics to cover the most likely organisms, and before leaving the clinic, should receive an intramuscular or IV dose of antibiotics. Antiemetics can be prescribed if nausea is a predominant symptom.

CASE CONTINUED

Because the patient appeared well, she was administered one dose of ceftriaxone intramuscularly, prescribed TMP/SMX for 21 days, with phone follow-up the next day, and a follow-up appointment with her PMD in one week. The urine was sent for culture and sensitivities and results were pending. Upon phone follow-up, however, the patient felt much worse, with increasing left-sided back pain, fever, nausea and now with several episodes of emesis. The patient was instructed to return to the clinic.

VS: Temp 39.8°C BP 146/94 HR 110 RR 20

PE: Appears in severe discomfort, constantly moving to obtain a comfortable position, retching occasionally, very warm. *HEENT:* dry mucous membranes. *Abdomen:* bowel sounds present, mild suprapubic tenderness, no peritoneal signs. *Back:* severe left costovertebral tenderness. Urine culture preliminary result – *Proteus.*

THOUGHT QUESTIONS

- What are possible causes for the patient's worsening clinical picture?
- What diagnostic studies or laboratory tests would you order?
- What would your management be now?

Possibilities for the worsening clinical picture include infected kidney stones or obstruction by a stone, a renal or perinephric abscess, emphysematous pyelonephritis, or an organism resistant to the antibiotic. The patient now has vital signs and physical examination suggesting bacteremia, dehydration, and intractable pain, thus warranting admission to the hospital for treatment and workup: CBC with differential, electrolyte panel including BUN and creatinine, blood cultures, and a UA with C&S; an IV should be started and broad-spectrum antibiotics should be administered with IV hydration and antiemetics. The preferred intravenous antibiotic regimen would be ampicillin with gentamycin – gentamycin is renally excreted and concentrates in the urine. Imaging studies are necessary. Although CT scans can miss smaller stones, it is the preferred imaging to determine whether an abscess or a stone is present. If an immediate CT scan cannot be obtained, a renal ultrasound would be a good option to detect hydronephrosis, suggesting obstruction, as well as an abscess. A plain abdominal film with a renal ultrasound can detect the majority of stones – approximately 85% of stones are radiopaque. (Only pure uric acid stones are radiolucent.) IVP and VCUG should be performed once the acute pyelonephritis is resolved.

QUESTIONS

145. Renal stones are most commonly composed of:
    A. Calcium phosphate
    B. Calcium oxalate
    C. Uric acid
    D. Struvite

146. An abdominal radiograph was obtained and is shown in Figure 37. This patient likely has a renal stone composed of:
    A. Calcium oxalate
    B. Uric acid
    C. Magnesium ammonium phosphate
    D. Cysteine

147. A patient with chronic pyelonephritis may develop all of the following complications EXCEPT:
    A. Hypertension
    B. Xanthogranulomatous pyelonephritis
    C. Renal abscess
    D. Focal glomerulosclerosis

148. Which organism classically manifests as sterile pyuria?
    A. Mycoplasma
    B. Ureaplasma
    C. Mycobacteria
    D. Serratia

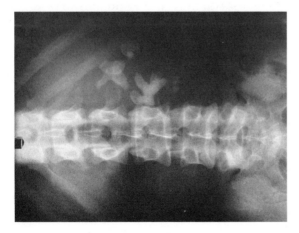

FIGURE 37 Abdominal radiograph. (Image courtesy of Raymond M. Hsu, MD, University of Hawai'i.)

CASE 38 / LOW BACK PAIN

ID/CC: EA is a 79-year-old African-American male who attends a clinic appointment complaining of low back pain.

HPI: EA is a thin African-American gentleman who is accompanied by his daughter. The daughter reports that EA has been complaining of low back pain for about six weeks, after stumbling over a throw rug, and landing on his bottom. He refused to come to the doctor, and has not seen a physician in 10 years, after his wife passed away from metastatic breast cancer. The daughter says, "I finally was able to drag him here today because the pain is not going away, and I had an appointment today." The patient takes acetaminophen for the pain, with only mild relief. The pain initially occurred with walking and sitting down, but now also occurs at night when lying down, without radiation.

PMHx: Mild hearing loss – hearing aids, presbyopia – bifocals, mild open-angle glaucoma, osteopenia, had been told in the past that he has an enlarged prostate

Meds: Acetaminophen as needed, timolol 0.25% one drop both eyes once a day

PSHx: None   **All:** NKDA   **FHx:** Noncontributory

SHx: Lives with one daughter, widower – wife died 10 years ago from metastatic breast cancer

ROS: No fever, chills, night sweats, nausea, vomiting, or diarrhea. Has mild nocturia and urinary hesitancy/frequency, without change in these symptoms for 10 years.

VS: Temp 36.7°C BP 144/88 HR 74 RR 16 Weight 50 kg

PE: Thin male, no acute distress. *Neck:* no midline tenderness. *CV:* RRR no murmurs. *Chest:* CTA bilaterally. *Abdomen:* benign. *Back:* lumbosacral spinal TTP, no paraspinal tenderness, negative straight leg raising, flexion/extension limited secondary to pain, no CVAT. *Rectal:* 2-cm firm, indurated, nontender nodule on the right lobe of the prostate. Guaiac negative, stool soft/brown. *Neurologic:* nonfocal, reflexes 2+ patellar bilaterally.

THOUGHT QUESTIONS
- What is the differential diagnosis for low back pain?
- What are the most likely diagnoses in this patient, and what would be the most concerning diagnosis?
- What studies would you order now?

It is helpful to think of low back pain in categories of etiology: musculoskeletal causes, systemic causes, and neurologic causes. Musculoskeletal causes are most common, including muscle strains, fractures, and osteoarthritis. Systemic causes include malignancy, metabolic bone disease (e.g., osteoporosis), and infectious etiologies (e.g., osteomyelitis). Neurologic causes include any neuropathy or demyelinating disease.

The most likely diagnosis in this patient is a vertebral fracture secondary to osteoporosis. The patient has a history of osteopenia, is thin, and fell on his sacrum – his past diagnosis of osteopenia may really be a diagnosis of osteoporosis, yielding a vertebral compression fracture. (Osteoporosis, however, is more common in postmenopausal women, Asians, Caucasians, smokers, those on chronic glucocorticoids, and those with sedentary lifestyles.) Another likely diagnosis, and one more concerning, is that of a pathologic vertebral fracture. This patient has a firm, indurated prostate nodule on DRE, and the first presentation of prostate cancer can be bony pain/metastases; most metastases from prostate cancer are to the axial skeleton.

Given the lengthy duration of the patient's back pain in conjunction with the prostate nodule, a workup for prostate cancer and bony metastases should be initiated. Blood tests, including a PSA, alkaline phosphatase, and serum calcium should be obtained. A plain lumbosacral radiograph can show vertebral fractures, and suggest bony metastases (the majority are osteolytic lesions). If bony metastasis is confirmed, a radionuclide bone scan should be anticipated. A referral to a urologist should be made for biopsy of the prostate nodule. CT scans, IV urography, and cystoscopy are not useful studies.

CASE CONTINUED

The patient had laboratory tests performed with the following results: PSA of 188 ng/ml (elevated), serum alkaline phosphatase level of 1132 (elevated), and an elevated serum calcium. A plain film of the lumbosacral spine reveals compression fractures of vertebrae L5-S2, with osteolytic lesions highly suggestive of bony metastases.

QUESTIONS

149. Which of the following medications acts by inhibiting the conversion of testosterone to dihydrotestosterone?
    A. Flutamide
    B. Finasteride
    C. Leuprolide
    D. Doxazosin

150. All of the following are screening tests for prostate cancer EXCEPT:
    A. Biopsy of a prostate nodule
    B. Digital rectal examination
    C. Serum prostate-surface antigen level
    D. Transrectal ultrasound of the prostate

151. All of the following factors in this patient's history could increase his fall risk EXCEPT:
    A. Throw rugs in the home
    B. Taking timolol for glaucoma
    C. Presbyopia
    D. Past history of osteopenia

152. The patient had a transrectal ultrasound-guided biopsy of the prostate nodule. The most likely histopathology expected is:
    A. Transitional cell carcinoma
    B. Clear cell carcinoma
    C. Adenocarcinoma
    D. Seminoma

CC/ID: 54-year-old hospitalized male with decreased urine output

HPI: FO is a 54-year-old homeless Caucasian male hospitalized for three days with right middle lobe community-acquired pneumonia. He defervesced over the last 24 hours with intravenous ceftriaxone, and is scheduled to be discharged in the morning. Overnight, however, the nursing staff notice that he has very little urine output: 100 cc for the 12-hour day shift. The house-officer is called to evaluate FO. He is asymptomatic and denies fever, chills, shortness of breath, chest pain, nausea, vomiting, diarrhea, dysuria, pain, or swelling of extremities. He informs the house-officer that the ibuprofen ordered for him two days ago really helped the pain with breathing or moving.

Review of the chart reveals:

PMHx: Significant only for CHF secondary to alcoholic dilated cardiomyopathy with an ejection fraction approximately 55%, and history of alcohol withdrawal seizures.

Meds: Ceftriaxone 1 g IV every 24 hours, ibuprofen 800 mg by mouth every eight hours, benazepril 40 mg by mouth daily, furosemide 40 mg by mouth twice a day, chlordiazepoxide 25 mg by mouth every eight hours, thiamine 100 mg by mouth once a day, folic acid 1 mg by mouth once a day, MVI 1 by mouth once a day, acetaminophen 650 mg by mouth every four hours as needed.

All: NKDA   **VS:** Afebrile BP 118/84 HR 64 RR 18 95% RA weight stable

PE: Exam essentially unchanged from admission. *Pertinent negatives:* moist mucous membranes, no JVD, RRR no murmurs, abdomen benign without suprapubic tenderness, no CVAT, no peripheral edema, skin without tenting, neurologic exam nonfocal, clear mentation. *Pertinent positives:* decreased breath sounds right middle field with rales, otherwise other fields clear – slightly improved since admission

---

THOUGHT QUESTION
- What should be done at this time to assess oliguria?

FO has been assessed for fluid status; he is euvolemic, with stable vital signs. A Foley catheter should be placed; urinary retention or obstruction is probable if urine output is more than 200 cc with catheter placement. A CBC with differential, serum sodium, potassium, chloride, CO_2, BUN, creatinine, glucose, calcium, magnesium, phosphorus, albumin, urinalysis with microscopy, urine osmolality, and urine electrolytes should be ordered. While laboratory data is pending, assess renal response to a fluid challenge. A conservative fluid challenge should occur in the patient with known CHF. The medication list should be reviewed for drugs that affect renal function.

CASE CONTINUED

A Foley catheter is placed with minimal urine output. A 250 cc normal saline fluid challenge yields a 50 cc urine output, which is sent for urinalysis, osmolality, sodium, and creatinine.

Serum electrolytes reveal: Na 135 (WNL), K 3.8 (WNL), Cl 118 (WNL), CO_2 27 (WNL), BUN 75 (elevated), Cr 2.5 (elevated). UA is normal, negative for protein/ketones/bilirubin/glucose/bacteria/RBC/WBC. Microscopy shows no casts, no cells, no organisms. UOsm 588 mOsm. Fractional excretion of sodium (FeNa) is calculated to be 3%. Other labs are within normal limits.

THOUGHT QUESTION
- Discuss the causes of acute renal failure. What is the cause of this patient's renal failure? What explains the high value of fractional excretion of sodium?

Acute renal failure occurs in 5% of hospitalized patients. It is divided into three classes of etiology: prerenal, renal (intrinsic), or postrenal.

Based on laboratory data and physical examination, the patient is likely in prerenal ARF. He has many predisposing factors for prerenal ARF: CHF, infection, diuretic use predisposing to hypovolemia, ACE-inhibitors, and NSAIDs. The patient does not exhibit any signs or symptoms of acute CHF, sepsis, or intravascular

TABLE 39. Etiology Divisions of Acute Renal Failure

	PRERENAL (60–70%)	RENAL (25–40%)	POSTRENAL (5–10%)

Cause	• Intravascular depletion
	  • Dehydration
	  • Hemorrhage
	  • Sepsis
	• Decreased circulating volume to kidneys
	  • CHF
	  • Cirrhosis
	  • Hepatorenal syndrome
	  • Nephrotic syndrome
	• Impaired renal blood flow
	  • ACE-inhibitors
	  • NSAIDs
		• Acute tubular necrosis (ATN)
		  • Ischemia
		  • Toxins
		• Glomerular disease
		  • Acute proliferative glomerulonephritis
		  • HIV-associated nephropathy
		  • Systemic lupus erythematosus
		  • Wegener's granulomatosis
		• Interstitial disease
		  • Pyelonephritis
		  • Allergic reactions
		  • Autoimmune disease
		• Micro- or macrovascular disease
			• Obstruction
			  • BPH
			  • Tumor
			  • Crystals
			  • Urethral stricture
			• Retention
			  • Bladder atony
			  • Neurogenic bladder

UA	Normal UA, possible concentrated urine, few hyaline casts	ATN—muddy brown granular casts, WBCs, mild proteinuria Glomerulonephritis—RBC casts, proteinuria Interstitial—WBCs, WBC casts, eosinophils, RBCs, proteinuria	Normal UA, few hyaline casts, possible RBCs
BUN:Cr ratio	>20:1	ATN—<20:1 Glomerulonephritis—>20:1 Interstitial—<20:1	>20:1
UOsm	>500	ATN—250–300 Glomerulonephritis – varies Interstitial – varies	<400
FeNa	<1%	ATN—>1% Glomerulonephritis—<1% Interstitial—varies	varies

depletion, making these causes less likely. He takes benazepril as an outpatient, making the ACE-inhibitor also less likely. The high-dose ibuprofen regiment (NSAID), however, is new, and has likely tipped his very fragile renal balance. High-dose NSAIDs in combination with ACE-inhibitors can diminish renal perfusion enough to cause ARF, especially in patients with delicate renal perfusion.

(ACE-inhibitors decrease the amount of angiotensin II; angiotensin II increases the GFR by constricting the efferent arteriole; decreased levels of angiotensin II lead to a dilated efferent arteriole with subsequent decreased glomerular filtration.)

(NSAIDs inhibit prostaglandin production; prostaglandin dilates the afferent arteriole, thereby increasing GFR; decreased levels of prostaglandin yield decreased GFR.)

The sodium is calculated by (serum creatinine × urine Na)/(serum Na × urine creatinine) × 100. It is not consistent with prerenal ARF in this patient, even though he is in prerenal ARF. This is secondary to furosemide, which increases urinary sodium excretion.

QUESTIONS

153. Which of the following statements regarding treatment for this patient is true?
    A. The patient's renal failure warrants emergent hemodialysis
    B. The patient should continue to receive ceftriaxone as ordered to treat pneumonia
    C. Furosemide should be discontinued
    D. Ibuprofen should be discontinued

154. Acute renal failure often leads to deranged metabolic studies. The main electrolyte imbalances are hyperkalemia and acidosis. Which of the following is not a treatment option for hyperkalemia?
    A. Albuterol nebulizer therapy
    B. Magnesium gluconate
    C. Hemodialysis
    D. Sodium bicarbonate
    E. Calcium carbonate

155. Which of the patient's medications requires adjusted dosing secondary to decreased metabolism in renal failure?
    A. Acetaminophen
    B. Thiamine
    C. Ceftriaxone
    D. Folic acid

156. Which of the following clinical scenarios requires emergent hemodialysis?
    A. An obtunded patient with COPD on two liters of oxygen, with an arterial blood gas revealing the following data: pH 7.21, pCO_2 88, pO_2 96
    B. An asymptomatic patient with a BUN of 58 and a creatinine of 4.5
    C. An adolescent female found unconscious with a suicide note and multiple empty bottles of aspirin next to her
    D. An asymptomatic patient with CHF on spironolactone who has a potassium level of 6.2, without EKG changes

CASE 40 / BLOODY DIARRHEA

ID/CC: DS is a 28-year-old Jewish female who presents to urgent care with two episodes of bloody diarrhea.

HPI: DS reports intermittent crampy abdominal pain for two days, with some loose, watery stools, but the bloody diarrhea started this evening, with two bloody stools and associated tenesmus. She notes some mucus in her stool. No nausea or vomiting. She thought her upset stomach might have been caused by some sushi she ate four days ago but says that her boyfriend ate the same thing and did not get sick. She takes magnesium aluminum hydroxide and loperamide over the counter, with only slight relief. She now feels slightly feverish, and is visibly worried. She went hiking about two weeks ago.

PMHx: Unremarkable   **PSHx:** None

Meds: Maalox as needed, loperamide as needed, oral contraceptives

All: NKDA   **FHx:** *Father:* hemorrhoids

SHx: Works as a financial analyst, enjoys camping and hiking, lives with her boyfriend

ROS: Above   **VS:** Temp. 38.0°C BP 124/68 HR 78 RR 16. *Weight:* 58 kg

PE: Worried female, no respiratory distress. *HEENT:* MMM, OP clear without lesions/erythema/exudate. *Skin:* warm, no rashes, no ecchymoses or petechiae, no pallor. *Abdomen:* BS present, severe tenderness to palpation in the left lower quadrant, no rebound, no guarding, no peritoneal signs. *Anoscopy:* grossly bloody, no hemorrhoids.

THOUGHT QUESTIONS

- What is the differential diagnosis for this presentation?
- What initial workup should be done for this patient?

There are many causes of bloody diarrhea. Any infection with invasive organisms, such as *Shigella*, enterotoxigenic *E. coli*, or *Entamoeba histolytica*, can cause bloody diarrhea. Any inflammatory state, such as Crohn's disease or ulcerative colitis, can cause this presentation, although Crohn's disease tends to present with nonbloody diarrhea. Vasculitis, cytotoxins, ischemia, and even coagulopathies are possible. Infectious and inflammatory etiologies are more likely in the febrile patient. Hemorrhoids are ruled out by anoscopy, and do not cause fever. It is unlikely that the sushi caused her symptoms, as toxin-mediated diarrhea is usually nonbloody, and occurs within 24 hours of ingestion. Hiking or camping could be a source for parasites, but the most frequent parasite would be *Giardia lamblia*, which causes nonbloody watery diarrhea.

The initial workup would include CBC with differential stool studies for ova and parasites, bacterial culture, and fecal leukocytes. If patient is severely dehydrated, serum electrolytes should be drawn.

CASE CONTINUED

DS had a hematocrit of 39, and a leukocytosis of 12 with 69% neutrophils. All other laboratory values were within normal limits. Her abdominal pain decreased, and no further episodes of bloody diarrhea occurred in the office. As she appeared nontoxic and well-hydrated, she was sent home with instructions not to take anti-diarrheal agents, to maintain a bland diet without caffeine or alcohol until her abdominal pain and diarrhea subsided, and to await stool results. She was instructed to return if the bloody diarrhea continued, the abdominal pain worsened, or she developed fever or chills.

A week later, the final stool studies showed no ova or parasites, many fecal leukocytes, no *Shigella*/*Salmonella*/enterotoxigenic *E. coli*. She was reassured with these results, until one month later when the symptoms recurred.

THOUGHT QUESTIONS
- What is the next step in diagnosis?
- What is the most likely diagnosis?

The next step in diagnosis would be to perform a flexible sigmoidoscopy to inspect for ulcerations and perform biopsies. Other important laboratory data would be a CBC (to recheck the hematocrit, platelets, leukocytosis), ESR (to determine inflammation), and a coagulation panel (to rule out any coagulopathies). A colonoscopy would not be indicated at this time, as any acute inflammation would increase the risk of perforation.

The patient likely has an acute colitis. Given her age and presenting symptoms, she probably has ulcerative colitis with mild disease.

QUESTIONS

157. Which of the following is NOT a complication of ulcerative colitis?
    A. Abscess formation
    B. Severe anemia
    C. Toxic megacolon
    D. Sclerosing cholangitis

158. Which of the following complications is more commonly found in Crohn's disease than in ulcerative colitis?
    A. Colon cancer
    B. Toxic megacolon
    C. Urolithiasis
    D. Severe anemia

159. Which dermatologic finding is an extraintestinal manifestation of inflammatory bowel disease?
    A. Erythema nodosum
    B. Rheumatoid nodules
    C. Erythema multiforme
    D. Erythema annulare

160. The following pathologic features are all found in ulcerative colitis EXCEPT:
    A. Submucosal inflammation
    B. Microabscesses in the crypts of Lieberkuhn
    C. Mucosal inflammation
    D. Skip lesions

CASE 41 / HEMATEMESIS

ID/CC: RO is a 63-year-old Caucasian man brought to the ED by ambulance after being found on the streets vomiting blood.

HPI: RO is a 63-year-old homeless male with PMHx significant for liver cirrhosis, who had been on a drinking binge for four days and started vomiting one day prior to presentation. He was visibly intoxicated in the ED, covered in blood, and responsive to questions. After stabilization in the ED, he was admitted to the inpatient service.

PMHx: Alcoholic liver cirrhosis, alcoholism, past admissions for GI bleeding

PSHx: None   **Meds:** None   **All:** NKDA   **FHx:** Unknown

SHx: Homeless, no tobacco/drugs, drinks two to three pints of liquor per day

ROS: No bright red blood per rectum, no weight changes, + easy bruising and bleeding, + melena starting the evening prior to admission, normal urination

VS: Temp 36.7°C BP 130/86 HR 104 RR 18

PE: *Gen:* intoxicated, talkative with slurred speech, blood stains on clothes. *Skin:* multiple spider angiomas on trunk. *HEENT:* PERRLA, EOMI, no nystagmus, dry OP. *Neck:* no JVD. *CV:* tachycardic, no murmurs. *Chest:* CTA bilaterally. *Abdomen:* nondistended, no caput, BS+, mild diffuse tenderness, no peritoneal signs, no organomegaly, no shifting dullness or fluid wave. *Rectal:* Guaiac +, black stool. *Neuro:* Nonfocal, reflexes 2+ biceps/patellar/Achilles without clonus, Babinski ↓ bilaterally

---

THOUGHT QUESTIONS

- What are the most likely causes of GI bleeding in this patient?
- What laboratory tests should be ordered?
- How should he be managed?

The most likely causes of upper GI bleeding (note hematemesis and melena indicating an upper GI source) in this alcoholic patient with liver cirrhosis are 1) ruptured esophageal varices secondary to likely portal hypertension, 2) Mallory-Weiss tears secondary to vigorous emesis and retching, 3) gastritis or peptic ulcer disease from alcohol intake, and 4) coagulopathy from impaired liver function.

Laboratory workup in the ED includes a CBC with platelets, coagulation panel with INR, LFTs, basic metabolic panel, and type and cross for the possibility of blood transfusion.

Management of the patient in the ED begins with assessing ABCs, obtaining intravenous access, performing a nasogastric aspirate to check for current bleeding, following the blood loss with serial hemoglobins and/or hematocrits, administering Vitamin K subcutaneously if the patient exhibits a coagulopathy, administering oral omeprazole if the patient can tolerate intake or IV Pepcid if not tolerating intake (only oral omeprazole has been proven to halt bleeding), and administering octreotide as the suspicion of esophageal varices is high. Fluid resuscitation via IVF should be started immediately, and blood transfusion if warranted; the patient may be premedicated with diphenhydramine and a minimal amount of acetaminophen before the transfusion. The patient should be admitted after ED management and stabilization.

CASE CONTINUED

The patient's upper GI bleeding was appropriately managed, and an upper esophagogastroduodenoscopy was scheduled for the next day. He continued to have a few episodes of hematemesis. Later on the evening of admission, the patient became severely agitated and confused. He was evaluated, and within the course of two hours was somnolent and minimally responsive.

PE on re-evaluation: Temp 37.0°C BP 120/80 HR 78 RR 16. *Gen:* moans to painful stimuli, unresponsive to questions. *HEENT:* eyes closed, do not open to stimuli; PERRLA, MMM. *Abdomen:* unchanged from admission. *Neuro:* withdraws to painful stimuli, no nystagmus, doll's eye movements intact, generalized hyperreflexia with multiple beats of clonus, Babinski equivocal.

QUESTIONS

161. On re-evaluation, the patient had a Glasgow coma score of:
    A. 2
    B. 7
    C. 9
    D. 12

162. What is the most likely explanation for the patient's deteriorating clinical condition?
    A. Spontaneous bacterial peritonitis
    B. Hepatorenal syndrome
    C. Hepatic encephalopathy
    D. Ischemic cerebrovascular accident

163. All of the following are physical findings present in a patient with end-stage liver cirrhosis EXCEPT:
    A. Caput medusae
    B. Telangiectasias
    C. Fetor hepaticus
    D. Hepatomegaly

164. All of the following are appropriate steps in intravenous fluid resuscitation EXCEPT:
    A. Placement of a femoral catheter
    B. Placement of two large bore peripheral catheters
    C. Infusion of normal saline
    D. Infusion of lactated Ringer's solution

ID/CC: A 42-year-old man comes to your drop-in clinic complaining of "the shakes."

HPI: TM is a patient of the Family Health Center, although he has been to only one-third of his scheduled appointments. He describes feeling depressed for the past three weeks due to the death of a close friend. He has been drinking "more vodka than usual" for the last two weeks; he has felt sick for the past 36 hours and hasn't had anything to eat or drink since then. Since last night he has felt very shaky; he vomited twice this morning.

PMHx: Borderline HTN; no medical treatment.   **Meds:** Occasional ibuprofen   **All:** NKDA

SHx: Lives alone in a single-room occupancy apartment building; family are across the country. Works odd jobs; currently delivering papers.

Alcohol: normally drinks one pint of vodka/day; recently upwards of five pints/day. Marijuana: occasional use. No other recreational drugs. No tobacco.

VS: Temp 38.6°C BP 165/100 HR 115 RR 20

PE: Very tremulous, agitated man; pacing around the room. *CV:* regular rhythm, tachycardic; midsystolic murmur at base. *Pulmonary:* CTA. *Abdomen:* soft, hyperactive bowel sounds; no hepatomegaly. *Rectal:* guaiac positive brown stool. *Extremities:* no C/C/E. *Neuro:* Reflexes 3+ throughout, symmetric, somewhat delirious.

THOUGHT QUESTIONS

- What additional history is important?
- What should your initial management be?
- How should you follow this patient's symptoms?

TM, by history and physical, is at significant risk for alcohol withdrawal syndrome. This syndrome displays the reverse of the depressive effects of alcohol: increased adrenergic, serotonergic, and cholinergic activity. You need to determine the exact frequency, amount, and timing of his drinking; past history of withdrawal or seizures, benzodiazepine use or other detoxification experiences. This patient with heme+ diarrhea, fever, tachycardia, and high risk for alcohol withdrawal syndrome needs to be admitted for further management. (Medically managed residential detoxification would be appropriate for a patient without the need for IV fluids or medicines.) Up to 70% of withdrawal patients have comorbid conditions such as infection, pancreatitis, GI bleed, or severe electrolyte abnormalities. Initially you should obtain IV access and begin aggressive hydration; order a basic metabolic panel, urine drug/toxicology screen, LFTs, CBC with differential, Ca, Mg, phosphate, and urine and blood cultures. You could consider an alcohol level if you doubt the history. You should give him thiamine, folate, and a multivitamin, then initiate your alcohol withdrawal treatment using the CIWA scoring system. (A standardized alcohol withdrawal assessment tool: see abbreviated CIWA scores below.)

1. Nausea and vomiting: None (0) to constant (7).
2. Tremor (observe with arms extended/fingers spread): None (0) to severe with flexed arms (7).
3. Paroxysmal sweats: None (0) to drenching (7).
4. Anxiety: None (0) to panic (7).
5. Agitation: Normal activity level (0) to pacing/thrashing (7).
6. Tactile disturbances: None (0) to continuous tactile hallucinations (7).
7. Auditory disturbances: Not present (0) to continuous auditory hallucinations (7).
8. Visual disturbances: Not present (0) to continuous visual hallucinations (7).
9. Headache: Not present (0) to extremely severe (7).
10. Orientation: Orientated, can do additions (0) to disorientated for place/person (4).

Add up the score: CIWA < 8 = No withdrawal, consider prophylaxis
                   CIWA 8–15 = Minor withdrawal
                   CIWA 16–25 = Moderate withdrawal
                   CIWA > 25 = Major withdrawal/delirium tremens

CASE CONTINUED

Your patient initially presents with a CIWA score of 18. He denies past seizures or withdrawal treatment. You treat him with 100 mg of chlordiazepoxide orally, believing that he is at least 36 hours out from his last drink. His lab tests show a magnesium of 1.4, and you begin IV repletion. His CIWA score one hour later is 25; he is yelling at anyone who walks into his room. What should your next step be?

This patient will fail oral treatment, and should be changed to intravenous withdrawal treatment. He needs to be transferred to a more intensive floor where he can get frequent checks. You should give him lorazepam IV bolus 2–4 mg as needed every 15–30 minutes to the desired sedation scale of 2–4.

TABLE 42. Sedation Scale	
1	Anxious/agitated
2	Cooperative
3	Response to command
4	Asleep, briskly responsive
5	Asleep, sluggishly responsive
6	Unresponsive

After six hours you can calculate the hourly drip rate according to the total lorazepam needed during the prior six hours, which can then be lowered by 25% each day as tolerated. After the dose of the drip is lowered to 1 mg per hour you can switch to chlordiazepoxide 150 mg by mouth every six hours. At this point your substance abuse counseling service can get more involved to start discussing outpatient rehabilitation options and long-term strategies.

QUESTIONS

165. Alcohol withdrawal seizures most commonly occur:
    A. 12 hours from the last drink
    B. Less than 48 hours from the last drink
    C. 72 hours from the last drink
    D. With a focal pattern

166. Which of the following benzodiazepines used for alcohol withdrawal may be given IM?
    A. Chlordiazepoxide
    B. Diazepam
    C. Lorazepam
    D. Valium

167. 25 mg of oral chlordiazepoxide is equivalent to how much lorazepam?
    A. 1–2 mg by mouth
    B. 4 mg IV
    C. 0.5 mg by mouth
    D. They work on different pathways

168. The mortality rate from major alcohol withdrawal (delerium tremens) is:
    A. 1%
    B. 5%
    C. 10%
    D. 20%

CASE 43 / AGITATION

ID/CC: JB is an 86-year-old Caucasian female in residence at a long-term-care nursing facility with agitation for one day.

HPI: The PMD is called to see JB at the nursing home. She has been agitated for one day, screaming and crying incoherently. She has tried to bite, hit, and scratch several care home staff members. Her behavior has been intermittent throughout the course of the day. At baseline, JB is usually reserved and cooperative, able to speak but usually not making any sense due to Alzheimer's dementia. Her behavior today is markedly changed. She is ambulatory at baseline, and although the nursing staff reports no falls, they have noticed that she has been unsteady on her feet. She has had no fevers, chills, or diarrhea, but she had two episodes of emesis and a decreased appetite. The staff is unable to comment on urinary symptoms because she is diapered for baseline incontinence.

PMHx: Alzheimer's dementia, osteoporosis – compression fractures C3, C4, C5; right femoral head fracture status post open reduction internal fixation eight years ago, urinary incontinence

Meds: Calcium carbonate 500 mg three times a day, Acetaminophen as needed   **All:** NKDA

SHx: Resident of long-term-care nursing facility for eight years after her hip fracture, previously lived with her son, who is her DPOA for health care, past occupation as a RN

Habits: No tobacco, alcohol, or other drugs

ROS: As noted in the HPI. Functional assessment from the medical chart reveals that the patient is unable to perform any ADLs or IADLs

THOUGHT QUESTION
- What are the differences between delirium and dementia?

TABLE 43. Differences Between Delirium and Dementia

	DELIRIUM	DEMENTIA
Onset	Acute	Chronic
Consciousness	Waxing and waning	Alert
Cognition	Disoriented/impaired	Disoriented
Speech pattern	Rapid or slowed; incoherent	Intelligible
Motor activity	Psychomotor agitation	Normal
Hallucinations	Auditory and visual	None
Prognosis	Reversible	Irreversible

CASE CONTINUED

VS: Temp 35.0°C rectal BP 120/72 HR 80 RR 18 O_2 Saturation 100% on RA

PE: *Gen:* thin female in no respiratory distress, in restraints, yelling. *Skin:* + skin tenting, dry, cool. *HEENT:* dry MMM, otherwise negative. *Neck:* no lymphadenopathy. *CV:* RRR no murmurs/gallops/rubs. *Chest:* CTA bilaterally, no rales. *Back:* no CVAT, no decubitus ulcers. *Abdomen:* BS present, soft, suprapubic tenderness to palpation, no peritoneal signs. *Genitourinary:* diapered, malodorous urine. *Ext:* WNL. *Neuro:* grossly nonfocal. *Mental Status:* oriented only to self, disoriented to place, time, and situation.

Labs: WBC 24.8/mm³ (Nl 4300–10,800), Hgb 12.6 g/dL (Nl 12–16), Hct 39% (Nl 37–48), Plts 253,000/mm³ (Nl 150,000–350,000), 93% neutrophils (Nl 60%), Na 160 (elevated), K 3.8 (WNL), Cl 110 (WNL), CO_2 17 (decreased), BUN 158 (elevated), Cr 3.7 (elevated), Gluc 130 (WNL), UA: dark yellow, 1.030, 1+ protein, 2+ occult blood, 3+ WBCs, 3+ ketones. Stat Gram stain of urine: many thick gram-negative rods, many PMNs, moderate RBCs. Urine culture pending

---

THOUGHT QUESTION

• What is the cause of the patient's delirium?

The patient has urosepsis, dehydration, and prerenal azotemia (acute renal failure). The urosepsis is characterized by hypothermia (a fever equivalent in the elderly), leukocytosis with a left shift, suprapubic tenderness, urinalysis with bacteria, and an increased anion gap metabolic acidosis (CO_2 17, anion gap of 33). The anion gap is calculated by ($Na - Cl - CO_2$). The acidosis is likely due to lactic acidosis and uremia. The mnemonic for etiologies of increased anion gap lactic acidosis is MUDPILERS: Methanol, Uremia, Diabetic ketoacidosis/starvation ketoacidosis/alcoholic ketoacidosis, Paraldehyde, INH and Iron toxicity, Lactic acidosis, Ethylene glycol, Rhabdomyolysis, Salicylates. Dehydration from decreased intake and increased output (polyuria from urinary infection and emesis) has caused a prerenal acute renal failure, evidenced by the BUN:Cr ratio > 20:1, hypernatremia suggestive of hemoconcentration, dry mucous membranes, and skin tenting.

QUESTIONS

169. The patient has a written advanced directive in her medical chart documenting her code status of DNR/DNI (Do Not Resuscitate/Do Not Intubate). Which of the following statements regarding treatment options is true?
    A. The patient should remain at the nursing home and receive analgesics and antipsychotics
    B. The patient should remain at the nursing home and receive only her current listed medications
    C. The patient should be transferred to the nearest hospice facility for comfort care
    D. The patient should be admitted to the nearest hospital for intravenous fluids and antibiotics

170. A functional assessment of an elderly person's activities of daily living includes inquiry about the patient's:
    A. Ability to perform household chores
    B. Ability to bathe oneself
    C. Ability to use the telephone
    D. Ability to prepare meals for oneself

171. What is the most common type of incontinence in elderly men and women?
    A. Urge incontinence
    B. Stress incontinence
    C. Overflow incontinence
    D. Functional incontinence

172. Which of the following interventions in the elderly is correctly paired with the level of prevention?
    A. Guidance on home safety for high-risk elderly – secondary prevention
    B. Smoking cessation and exercise counseling in the elderly – secondary prevention
    C. Pneumococcal vaccination at age 65 – primary prevention
    D. Colorectal cancer screening with colonoscopy every 10 years after age 50 – primary prevention

CASE 44 / OBESITY

ID/CC: A 45-year-old Caucasian woman presents to your clinic for regular healthcare. She says: "You've gotta help me lose some weight!"

HPI: CC describes herself as a healthy, active woman. She has been trying to lose weight since she was 10 years old. She has tried "every diet in the tabloids," but always ends up five to 10 pounds heavier at the end. She exercises by walking three times a week for about 30 minutes. She also hikes on the weekends.

PMHx: Noncontributory **PSHx:** None **Meds:** Nutritional weight loss supplement

All: NKDA **FHx:** Sister with ovarian cancer

SHx: Lives alone, works as assistant at bank. Smokes occasional cigarettes at parties. No alcohol or other drugs.

VS: BP 135/88 HR 73 Height 5'6" (168 cm) Weight 256 pounds (116 kg)

PE: *HEENT:* MMM, sclera anicteric, thyroid nonpalpable. *CV:* distant heart sounds; no M/R/G heard. *Pulmonary:* CTA. *Abdomen:* NABS, nontender, nondistended. *Extremities:* no C/C/E. *Skin:* Mild erythema/flaking in breast folds bilaterally.

THOUGHT QUESTIONS

- What other key points in the history and physical do you need to discover?
- What medical conditions occur with higher frequency in obese people?
- What are effective interventions to pursue in this patient?

This patient has made your job easier by bringing up her obesity in a direct manner. Many obese patients will never introduce the topic due to many different obstacles (which can include the value judgments of physicians and clinic equipment that may not accommodate their large size). Start by taking a weight and diet history, *** prior attempted weight-loss strategies. Ask about eating disorder behaviors. Take a thorough social history including history of isolation, harassment, or abuse. Ask about seatbelt use and access to public places for the morbidly obese. Accept that weight loss may not be possible for many patients—you can still help them as their doctor. Obese patients are at increased risk for hypertension, hyperlipidemia, diabetes, coronary artery disease, sleep apnea, degenerative joint disease, depression, nonalcoholic steatohepatosis, and cancers: cervical, breast, endometrial, and ovarian. These conditions need to be screened for and treated regardless of the patient's size. It is appropriate to weigh people privately. Interventions for obesity should be recommended carefully.

- Low-fat, high-fiber diets with moderate caloric values are best.
- Goal weight loss should be no more than eight pounds per month.
- Add things (vegetables, fruits, fibers) rather than take things away.
- Exercise in a sustainable, reasonable manner: chair exercise is better than no exercise.
- Even low amounts of sustained weight loss (5–10%) can have significant impact on health and quality of life.
- Commercial weight-loss businesses are costly and may not achieve lasting weight loss.
- Pharmacologic treatment should be approached cautiously.
- Surgical intervention should be reserved for severely obese individuals (>100% overweight or BMI >40) who have failed more conservative therapy. The most common surgical options are Roux-en-Y gastric bypass and vertically banded gastropexy (stapling). These achieve a higher degree of weight loss than dietary or drug treatments (30–45 kg in most patients), have low mortality (1/700), but have approximately 5% morbidity (usually infection) and 2–7% reoperation rate.

CASE CONTINUED

Your patient reveals that she hasn't had a Pap smear for five years, and that she has had some lower abdominal pain occasionally, unrelated to her irregular menstrual cycles. After her Pap smear, you perform a pelvic exam in which her ovaries are not palpable. You prescribe her with clotrimazole cream to treat her mild tinea under her breasts and recommend a more supportive bra. You schedule her for a pelvic ultrasound to evaluate her ovaries due to the combination of lower abdominal pain, family history of ovarian cancer, and a body habitus that excludes a sensitive exam of pelvic organs.

QUESTIONS

173. What is this patient's body mass index (BMI)?
    A. 27
    B. 35
    C. 41
    D. 50

174. What percentage of U.S. women have a BMI of 25 or above?
    A. 10
    B. 25
    C. 35
    D. 55

175. The loss of one pound of fat requires caloric deficit of:
    A. 1000 calories
    B. 2500 calories
    C. 3500 calories
    D. 5000 calories

176. What is the only pharmacologic therapy listed below that may be safe and efficacious for the treatment of obesity?
    A. Sibutramine
    B. Dexfenfluramine
    C. Fenfluramine
    D. Phenylpropanolamine

ID/CC: A 55-year-old Caucasian man presents to your clinic to get "that colon cancer test."

HPI: RH is an active man who hasn't been to a doctor since he was 40; "I didn't need to go." One of his colleagues at work recently had a colonoscopy and described it in detail; your patient feels that he should get his "tubes checked out."He denies any problems of constipation, diarrhea, or stool changes.

PMHx: Knee arthroscopy for torn ACL age 40, occasional migraine headaches

Meds: Aspirin "one a day," vitamin E

All: NKDA   **FHx:** Mother died of breast cancer age 67, no colon cancer or polyps in family

Habits: Drinks one to two mixed drinks per night; no tobacco or other drugs

Diet Hx: Eats two meals/day with red meat; one serving of vegetables/day

---

THOUGHT QUESTIONS

• What is the overall risk and prevalence of colon cancer?

• What is this patient's risk of colorectal cancer?

• What are the different options for colon cancer screening?

Colorectal cancer is the third most common malignancy in the developed world, and the second leading cause of death in North America. Without screening or preventive therapy, 1 in 17 Americans will develop colorectal cancer. Incidence of colorectal cancer depends on the presence or absence of identifiable risk.

TABLE 45-1. Percent of All Colorectal Cancers by Risk Category

Average risk (no identifiable risk factor)	75%
Family history of colorectal cancer	15–20%
Hereditary nonpolyposis colorectal cancer	3–8%
Familial adenomatous polyposis	1%
Ulcerative colitis	1%

This patient, as he has no identifiable risk factor, would be in the sporadic case or average risk category, although his carnivorous diet does increase his risk somewhat. Options for colon cancer screening include combinations of all of the following: fecal-occult blood testing (three serial tests for blood in the stool), flexible sigmoidoscopy (direct visualization to the splenic flexure), double-contrast barium enema, and colonoscopy (with real-time biopsy potential).

CASE CONTINUED

Your patient, although he is very interested in getting a colonoscopy, is willing to listen to other options. You attempt to explain fecal occult blood testing and the differences between flexible sigmoidoscopy and colonoscopy. You explain that FOBT is a screening test only, with the follow-up test being either a sigmoidoscopy or colonoscopy, depending on the result. Also, a colonoscopy is indicated post sigmoidoscopy if any polyp is found (occurs 25% of the time). Colonoscopy is the only way to obtain a biopsy at the time of test. Barium enema is a less commonly used screening method. Your patient's insurance will only cover FOBT and sigmoidoscopy for low-risk screening; colonoscopy is covered for positive FOBT results. Your patient wants to pay out of pocket for the colonoscopy so he can skip the other options. You inform him of the complication rates (1/1000 perforation risk, 2/1000 hemorrhage risk, 1/10,000 mortality) and refer him to the gastroenterologist for his exam.

THOUGHT QUESTIONS
- How are sensitivity, specificity, positive predictive value, and negative predictive value calculated?
- What are the drawbacks of a very sensitive test?

TABLE 45-2. Sensitivity, Specificity, Positive Predictive Value, and Negative Predictive Value

		DISEASE STATE	
		Present	Absent
Test Result	Positive	A (true positives)	B (false positives)
	Negative	C (false negatives)	D (true negatives)

Sensitivity (the proportion of people with disease who have a positive test) = A/(A + C)

Positive predictive value (probability of disease in a patient with a positive test) = A/(A + B)

Specificity (proportion of people without disease who have a negative test) = B/(B + D)

Negative predictive value (probability of not having the disease with a negative test) = D/(C + D)

There is usually a trade-off between sensitivity and specificity. A very sensitive test will usually confer more false positives; a sensitive test is most helpful when the probability of the disease is low.

Prevalence= (A + C)/(A + B + C + D)

The predictive value, a more important value when interpreting the results of an individual patient's test, is dependent on the prevalence of the disease being tested. As the prevalence approaches zero, the positive predictive value gets very small.

QUESTIONS

177. The sensitivity for detection of cancer or a large bleeding polyp of the Hemoccult II test (three serial FOBT with Hemoccult developer) is closest to:
    A. 90%
    B. 75%
    C. 50%
    D. 25%

178. The specificity of the fecal occult blood test will be _____ by the ingestion of red meat, aspirin, turnips, horseradish, and vitamin C for two days before or during the sampling.
    A. Increased
    B. Decreased
    C. Not affected
    D. It is impossible to say without knowing the size of the patient population

179. Screening with flexible sigmoidoscopy followed by colonoscopy for a positive test catches what percentage of all advanced neoplasms?
    A. 30%
    B. 40%
    C. 50%
    D. 70–80%

180. Which of the following is false regarding colon cancer screening?
    A. If chosen as the screening method, screening colonoscopy should be performed every five years
    B. Double-contrast barium enema detects 50–70% of polyps in the colon
    C. Currently, only 10–30% of Americans over age 50 have any type of screening for colon cancer
    D. Fecal-occult blood testing, sigmoidoscopy, double-contrast barium enema, and colonoscopy are all equally "cost-effective" as screening strategies

CASE 46 / TRISOMY 21

ID/CC: A 49-year-old Caucasian woman with Down syndrome presents to your office for primary care.

HPI: DP is a high-functioning woman accompanied by her home health nurse. She has only had emergency care for the past two years due to insurance issues. She has been feeling well and she has no complaints. Her nurse notes that she seems to be "slowing down" a little, that she is quite sleepy during the day and nods off sometimes at work. No one sleeps in her room, although her neighbors note that sometimes they can hear her snore through the walls.

PMHx: s/p VSD repair age 10 months, partial hearing loss; wears hearing aids

Meds: Multivitamin **All:** NKDA

SHx: Lives in assisted living facility with two hours of care from home health nurse. Parents are still alive and visit weekly. She works in an art studio for the developmentally disabled. No DPOA (durable power of attorney).

THOUGHT QUESTIONS

- What are the primary care needs of this patient?
- What special screening tests are indicated in this patient?
- What role can the primary care provider play?

Adults with Down syndrome qualify for all usual preventative screening, as well as some additional tests. Sexually active women need an annual Pap; for a non-sexually active woman who refuses Pap smear, a bimanual exam with finger directed cytology is recommended. For the patient who refuses pelvic exam, an ultrasound or exam under sedation can be considered. If the patient needs examinations or procedures such as a dental extraction, other indicated healthcare maintenance can be done at the same time, with consent. The primary care provider can be instrumental in helping the family address advance directives, estate planning, and power of attorney. Most often, conservatorship (granting healthcare decision-making power to someone other than the patient) is not indicated for patients with Down syndrome, as they are usually competent to make life decisions. The primary care provider is also essential during acute illness to help provide information about baseline functioning and health. Behavior change or decline in function may be the only clue to an underlying illness.

The special screening tests indicated in this patient are:

1. Thyroid function test screening (annually). Hypothyroidism occurs in 10–40% of adults with Down syndrome.
2. Neurological exam to evaluate for cord compression (due to increased ligamentous laxity—annually). 14% of adults with Down syndrome have atlanto-axial instability; anesthesiologists need to be especially careful during intubation.
3. Audiologic exam/evaluation of hearing aid function (every two years); hearing loss occurs in up to 70% of Down syndrome patients.
4. Eye exam (biannually); increased incidence of cataracts.
5. Screen for symptoms of diabetes; consider blood test.
6. Mental status/functioning assessment.
7. Dental assessment: Increased periodontal disease and gingivitis.
8. Sleep history: Obstructive sleep apnea is present in approximately half of Down syndrome patients; it may be related to obesity or hypotonia.

CASE CONTINUED

Your patient is not sexually active, but agrees to a pelvic exam. Her physical exam is notable for a normal oxygen saturation, mildly elevated BP at 145/85, and clear lungs.

THOUGHT QUESTIONS
- What tests should you order now?
- What treatment options are available if this patient does have sleep apnea?

In addition to a screening TSH, this patient clearly needs a sleep study to assess for possible apnea. Usually the symptoms of daytime hypersomnolence and complaints by the bed partner of snoring and interrupted breathing would trigger an investigation of sleep apnea. However, in patients with other mental disabilities, a mild decline in functioning may be the only indication of sleep apnea. Apnea is defined as the cessation of ventilation due to any mechanism. Obstructive sleep apnea is caused by collapse of the pharyngeal walls and closure of the upper airway. The upper limit of normal for apneic episodes is between 10 and 20 per hour; however, these brief pauses should not cause a drop in oxygen saturation. A sleep study is a formal polysomnographic study that includes continuous oxygen saturation monitoring and respiration tracing. Treatment of sleep apnea involves weight loss and a continuous positive airway pressure mask (keeping the pharynx open throughout the respiratory cycle) for nighttime use. Surgical intervention is warranted if the condition is severe and does not improve with conservative measures. Dental devices and pharmacologic therapies are less widely used.

QUESTIONS

181. In order to assess this patient's cardiac function, she needs:
    A. An echocardiogram
    B. A Holter monitor
    C. Careful cardiac auscultation
    D. An exercise treadmill test

182. Behavioral changes in an adult with Down syndrome may be due to:
    A. Hearing loss
    B. Hypothyroidism
    C. Obstructive sleep apnea
    D. Major depression
    E. All of the above

183. The most common neuropsychiatric complication in adults aging with Down syndrome is:
    A. Alzheimer's dementia
    B. Depression
    C. Autism
    D. Obsessive-compulsive disorder

184. Seizures, with an incidence rate of 5–10% in patients with Down syndrome, occur most commonly in which of the following age groups:
    A. Infancy
    B. The first decade
    C. Teenagers
    D. Over age 60

CASE 47 / CHECKUP

ID/CC: KN is a 63-year-old Vietnamese male recently immigrated to the United States who presents to the clinic for a checkup.

HPI: The patient moved to the United States six months ago to live with his children. He has no complaints at this time.

PMHx: Borderline HTN   **Meds:** Herbal medicine for sporadic aches and pains   **All:** NKDA

FHx: Father died at age 79 years from a stroke. Mother died at age 84 years from "old age"

SHx: Lives with one son and one daughter, their spouses, and three grandchildren. Widower – wife died from pneumonia in Vietnam years ago. Currently unemployed, was a factory-worker in Vietnam

Habits: One pack per day tobacco for 40 years. No alcohol, no drugs

ROS: Has a dry cough off and on for several years, otherwise denies any fever, chills, night sweats, stool changes, melena, bright red blood per rectum, or weight loss. KN notes that the adjustment to the United States is difficult, but he is happy to be with his children and grandchildren especially since he and his wife had many difficulties bearing children – they had a total of five miscarriages.

VS: Afebrile BP 144/96 HR 70 RR 18 100% RA

PE: Normal physical examination except for the rectal examination which is positive for occult blood.

A number of screening labs are sent, all of which are within normal limits, except for a hemoglobin of 10.8 g/dL, and a hematocrit of 35%, with a mean corpuscular volume (MCV) of 75 fL.

THOUGHT QUESTIONS

- What is the differential diagnosis for microcytic anemia?
- What further workup should be done for this patient's microcytic anemia?

Anemia is classified into three broad categories based upon red blood cell appearance and indices, specifically the mean corpuscular volume (MCV): macrocytic anemia (MCV > 100 fL), normocytic anemia (MCV 80–100 fL), and microcytic anemia (MCV < 80 fL).

TABLE 47. Differential Diagnosis of Microcytic Anemia

TYPE OF MICROCYTIC ANEMIA	MECHANISM
Iron deficiency	• Increased requirements (e.g., pregnancy) • Poor intake • Decreased absorption • Chronic blood loss
Anemia of chronic disease	• Decreased RBC lifespan • Unresponsive bone marrow • Inability to utilize iron stores
Thalassemia	• Defective synthesis of alpha-chain subunit of hemoglobin (alpha-thalassemia) • Defective synthesis of beta-chain subunit of hemoglobin (beta-thalassemia)
Sideroblastic anemia	• Ineffective erythropoiesis (due to toxins like lead or alcohol)
Other hemoglobinopathies	• E.g., sickle-cell

Based upon the MCV, this patient has a microcytic anemia; a peripheral smear should still be examined, however, to assess RBC appearance. Mentzer's index can be calculated to attempt to distinguish between iron deficiency anemia and thalassemia. Mentzer's index is calculated as the MCV/RBC; a value less than 13 favors thalassemia, while more than 13 favors iron deficiency. In addition, the serum iron and ferritin levels should be ordered. A total iron binding capacity (TIBC) can be added as well. In the patient who is older than 50 years old, with an anemia and hemoccult positive stool, a screening colonoscopy is also included to assess for occult GI malignancy.

CASE CONTINUED

Peripheral smear: 2+ hypochromia, 2+ microcytosis. Mentzer's index = 10. Serum iron: normal. Serum ferritin: normal. TIBC: normal. Colonoscopy reveals no polyps or abnormalities to the right colon, internal hemorrhoids are present.

The workup rules out iron deficiency, anemia of chronic disease, and sideroblastic anemia. To assess the possibility of thalassemia, a hemoglobin electrophoresis is ordered. Results show a decreased hemoglobin A2.

QUESTIONS

185. What type of thalassemia does this patient have?
    A. Beta-thalassemia minor
    B. Beta-thalassemia major
    C. Alpha-thalassemia trait
    D. Alpha-thalassemia silent carrier state

186. Which of the following statements regarding alpha-thalassemia is true?
    A. Hemoglobin Bart's is composed of a tetramer of beta chains
    B. Hemoglobin H is composed of a tetramer of gamma chains
    C. Heinz bodies are intracellular inclusions formed by the precipitation of hemoglobin H
    D. Exchange transfusion is a treatment modality for hemoglobin Bart's

187. Which of the following is not a sign or symptom of beta-thalassemia major?
    A. Chipmunk facies
    B. Hepatomegaly
    C. Small spleen
    D. Pallor

188. Which of the following is not a treatment modality for beta-thalassemia major?
    A. Ferrous sulfate
    B. Splenectomy
    C. Blood transfusion
    D. Bone marrow transplantation

ID/CC: A 50-year-old Caucasian man comes to your clinic to establish primary care.

HPI: RL is "feeling his age," but has no specific complaints. He describes himself as a relatively healthy man. He complains of feeling a little low energy, but no shortness of breath or chest pain. He had a blood pressure taken at a health fair two weeks ago that was 150/95: "Is that bad, doctor?"

ROS: Describes his mood as good. Sleeps well. Occasional urinary hesitancy; no sexual dysfunction.

PMHx: Arthroscopic repair of torn ACL age 32, otherwise none.

Meds: Takes multivitamin, occasional famotidine over-the-counter.   **All:** NKDA

FHx: Father died of stroke age 71, mother (age 78) with HTN. Sister with breast cancer s/p mastectomy.

SHx: Investment banker, lives with wife and two children ages 15 and 13. Nonsmoker. Drinks one to two glasses red wine per night. Plays basketball with friends on the weekends.

VS: BP 140/85 HR 75 RR 14 Height 5'11", Weight 230 pounds

PE: *General:* moderately overweight. *HEENT:* small pterygium left eye; sclera anicteric; EOMI, PERRLA. *Neck:* no LAN; no JVD. Carotid upstroke normal bilaterally; no bruits. *CV:* RR, rate at 75. No M/R/G. PMI at mid-clavicular line. *Pulmonary:* CTA; no crackles or wheezes. *Abdomen:* soft, NABS. No HSM. *Genitourinary:* no testicular masses. *Rectal:* normal tone, prostate smooth and nontender, symmetric; no masses palpated. *Extremities:* no C/C/E. *Neuro:* nonfocal. *Skin:* few scattered atypical nevi, flaking on naso-labial folds.

THOUGHT QUESTIONS
- What should be included in the primary care of this patient?
- What testing and follow-up care are indicated?

Primary care of a 50-year-old male should begin with a detailed personal and family history and a detailed physical exam. Physical exam should include weight and visual acuity. Immunizations to consider for this healthy 50-year-old man: tetanus booster (if more than 10 years since prior) and influenza vaccine if the patient requests. Routine screening tests could include a prostate specific antigen, but only after an informed discussion of risks/benefits of testing and the false positive/false negative rates. (Screening asymptomatic, low-risk males for prostate cancer has not been shown to improve morbidity or mortality from the disease; many unnecessary and painful follow-up procedures result.) Colon cancer screening should be discussed, and fecal occult blood testing ordered followed by flexible sigmoidoscopy (or colonoscopy if indicated). Risk of tuberculosis should be assessed; consider a PPD placement. Detailed sexual history should be obtained to assess risk of STDs including HIV. This patient most likely will have hypertension, so routine laboratory tests of this patient should include: urinalysis, CBC, basic metabolic panel, and fasting lipid profile. You may consider a TSH, given his complaint of fatigue. A baseline EKG is indicated.

CASE CONTINUED

Your patient is cooperative with your plan and happy to finally be under the care of a physician. You discuss his possible high blood pressure and options for interventions. He comes back in two weeks to discuss the results of his tests. His blood pressure today is 170/90. *Urinalysis:* normal. *CBC:* normal. *BMP:* normal. *Fasting lipids:* total cholesterol 221 LDL 150 HDL 51 TG 100 (Note: all cholesterol levels in mg/dL)

TABLE 48. Medication Classes for the Treatment of Hyperlipidemia

NAME	INDICATIONS	EFFECTS	SIDE EFFECTS
Bile acid sequestrants	High LDL	Lower LDL, minimal change HDL	Constipation, heartburn, bloating
Niacin (nicotinic acid)	High LDL, low HDL	Lower LDL, raise HDL, lower TG	Flushing, itching, ulcer, rash
Gemfibrozil	High TG	Lower TG, raise HDL	Interacts with warfarin
Probucol	High LDL	Lower LDL, lower HDL	Diarrhea, lowers HDL
HMG Co-A reductase inhibitors	High LDL	Lower LDL, minor raise HDL	Increased transaminases, myositis

QUESTIONS

189. This patient's estimated 10-year risk of coronary artery disease is approximately:
    A. 3%
    B. 8%
    C. 15%
    D. 28%

190. What is this patient's goal LDL?
    A. <160
    B. <130
    C. <100
    D. As low as it can go

191. Goal LDL is <100 for patients with all of the following EXCEPT:
    A. Nephrotic syndrome
    B. Diabetes
    C. Abdominal aortic aneurysm
    D. Symptomatic carotid artery disease

192. This patient's intervention may include all of the following EXCEPT:
    A. Step I American Heart Association diet
    B. Step II American Heart Association diet
    C. Pharmacologic lipid-lowering therapy
    D. Increased red wine intake

CASE 49 / LOW ENERGY

ID/CC: A 46-year-old Caucasian woman comes to her regularly scheduled Pap appointment complaining of feeling "low energy."

HPI: LM is generally somewhat anxious and schedules appointments about every three months. She describes for the past month or so feeling generally tired; that it is difficult for her to go about her daily activities. Her last menstrual period was one week late and unusually heavy. She has gained five pounds in the last two months. She denies depressed mood, and has maintained a normal level of interest in her daily activities.

ROS: Usually regular menstrual cycles, birth control method: husband with vasectomy. Normal lipid levels six months prior.

PMHx: 1. Treated LGSIL. 2. Bunion surgery   **Meds:** Calcium   **All:** NKDA

FHx: Sister with rheumatoid arthritis   **VS:** BP 125/80, HR 75, RR 16

PE: *HEENT:* MMM, PERRLA, sclera anicteric, normal conjunctiva. *Neck:* no thyromegaly/nodules. *CV:* RRR, no M/R/G. *Pulmonary:* CTA. *Extremities:* no C/C/E. *Neuro:* Reflexes 2+, slightly delayed relaxation phase.

THOUGHT QUESTIONS

- What are possible reasons for this patient's fatigue?
- What other points in the history should you ask?
- What further evaluation would be warranted at this point?

Fatigue is one of the most common complaints encountered in primary care visits, and can be challenging to address. The differential is broad, and could encompass almost every medical diagnosis. The major categories to think of are: psychological (depression, anxiety), pharmacologic, endocrine (hypothyroidism, diabetes), neoplastic, hematologic (anemia), infectious, cardiopulmonary, connective tissue disease, and disturbed sleep. A detailed history can help clarify which route to investigate more thoroughly. Ask about all of the somatic manifestations of depression, nervousness; investigate sources of stress, as well as alcohol, recreational drugs, and sleeping assists. Check for history of fever, adenopathy, polyuria, cold intolerance, and joint pain, as well as symptoms of sleep apnea, gastroesophageal reflux disease, and allergies. In this patient with clues of heavy menstrual cycle, weight gain, and slightly abnormal reflexes, a thyroid function test is indicated, as well as a CBC to evaluate for anemia.

CASE CONTINUED

LM is relieved to have a blood test and agrees to return in three days to discuss the results. You receive her results: TSH 25.6 mU/L (nl. 0.4-4.4) WBC 8.5 Hct 40.1 MCV 85 Plts. 210. You call the lab and ask them to add on a free T4 measurement to the initial blood draw, which returns with a "low-normal" value.

THOUGHT QUESTIONS
- What do you tell your patient now?
- What medical treatment is indicated?
- What further workup does she need?

Your patient has overt hypothyroidism and needs thyroid hormone repletion. It is a relatively common diagnosis, with an annual incidence in women over 40 of approximately 0.2%. It is usually not possible to identify the underlying etiology, although the most common cause is auto-immune thyroiditis or Hashimoto's thyroiditis (also called chronic lymphocytic thyroiditis). Patients with Hashimoto's may initially be hyperthyroid but always progress to hypothyroidism. You should ask about neck radiation, recent viral illness, previous Lithium therapy, neck or pituitary surgery, and recent pregnancy. Palpate the patient's neck again, checking for tenderness (found with subacute thyroiditis—usually postviral), enlargement (early Hashimoto's disease, postpartum patients, iodide deficiency), or nodularity (late Hashimoto's). Antimicrosomal antibodies could be ordered to confirm the diagnosis of Hashimoto's thyroiditis. Replacement therapy with thyroxine is necessary to restore your patient's normal metabolic state. The starting dose of her medicine should be 50 micrograms of levothyroxine per day; you can increase in 25 to 50 microgram increments every four weeks. The dose normally needed is 1.7 mcg/kg body weight per day. She should begin to feel better in three to four weeks.

QUESTIONS

193. When should this patient's labs be checked again, and what should you order?
    A. TSH and FT4 two weeks after starting therapy
    B. FT4 in two weeks and TSH in six weeks
    C. TSH and FT4 in two months
    D. TSH only in six weeks

194. All of the following are possible side effects of excessive thyroid replacement therapy except:
    A. Worsening coronary artery disease
    B. Hyperlipidemia
    C. Osteoporosis
    D. Palpitations

195. A different patient, a 65-year-old woman, returns to discuss the results of her screening TSH (which was 8.5 mU/L). You:
    A. Tell her she has hypothyroidism and immediately start her on levothyroxine
    B. Tell her she has hyperthyroidism
    C. Tell her that her thyroid function is normal for now
    D. Tell her that she has subclinical hypothyroidism

196. U.S. Preventive Services Task Force guidelines currently recommend:
    A. Against general thyroid testing of the population, and do not recommend for or against mass screening of older patients
    B. Screening for thyroid function in all postpartum patients and all women over the age of 50
    C. Screening for thyroid function periodically in women over age 35 and men over age 50
    D. Against all thyroid function test screening

CASE 50 / "I CAN'T TAKE MY MEDICINES"

ID/CC: A 45-year-old Latino man comes to his appointment complaining of belly pain and nausea: "I can't take my medicines."

HPI: EB is patient in your clinic and has a prior diagnosis of type 2 diabetes mellitus. He has been feeling increasingly nauseated with belly pain for the past two months, especially immediately after taking his "sugar pills." He also has been getting headaches and urinating more at night. He denies fever or chills; he does have occasional diarrhea (non-bloody). EB thinks that the pills are hurting him, and he has been taking them irregularly. He does not have a working glucometer at his house.

PMHx: 1. Type 2 DM diagnosed age 40; no known end-organ damage. Last Hgb A1C 15 months ago: 7.8. (normal under 6.0). 2. BPH.

Meds: 1. ASA 325 mg qd. 2. Acarbose 50 mg tid. 3. Glipizide 10 mg qd.

All: NKDA   **FHx:** Mother recently diagnosed with metastatic ovarian cancer, sister with DM.

SHx: Lives with extended family, also now caring for mother in home with hospice assistance. Does not drink; smokes one or two cigarettes when he "needs" to.

VS: BP 130/85 HR 85 RR 16 afebrile

PE: Heavy gentleman, no distress. *HEENT:* MMM, sclera anicteric. *CV:* RRR no M/R/G. *Pulmonary:* CTA. *Abdomen:* obese, soft, nontender to palpation, NABS. *Extremities:* no C/C/E; feet without lesions. *Neuro:* Reflexes 2+, nonfocal.

THOUGHT QUESTIONS

- What should you do next while this patient is still in the office?
- What factors could be contributing to his complaints?
- What type of follow-up should this patient have?

EB is presenting to you at a crucial time in his life: his health is deteriorating, he is dealing with a devastating situation at home, and he has come to you for help. This is an ideal time for intervention! His healthcare has clearly been slipping through the cracks given his most recent Hgb A1C of 15 months ago. It is somewhat unclear from his story which came first, but he seems to be having both side effects from his medication (likely the acarbose) and symptoms of hyperglycemia. (Hypoglycemia, which is possible but rare in a patient taking a sulfonylurea, would cause dizziness, tachycardia, and waning consciousness.) He needs an immediate blood glucose measurement and a urine dipstick. He should have complete laboratory studies including basic metabolic panel, liver function tests, fasting lipid panel, hemoglobin A1C, and urine for microalbuminuria screening. Goals for today's visit should include close follow-up with utilization of the diabetes educators in your clinic, possibly a home health visit as well.

CASE CONTINUED

EB's FSBG is 280 (three hours post-prandial). His urine shows 3+ glucose but no leukoestrase. You ask him to continue glipizide but discontinue the acarbose and return in four days for the results of his laboratory testing. His results are: normal LFTs and BMP; LDL 150, HDL 40, total cholesterol 240; Hgb. A1C 12.2. You start him on one new medicine and schedule him for follow-up in one week with the diabetes educator and in two weeks with you.

THOUGHT QUESTIONS

- What are the differences among the different oral medicines for type 2 DM?
- What medicine would you choose?

TABLE 50. Medications for Type 2 Diabetes Mellitus

MEDICATION	MECHANISM OF ACTION	DOSE	SIDE EFFECTS	CONTRAINDICATIONS	MONITORING	EXPECTED REDUCTION Hgb A1C
Repaglinide (meglitinides)	Stimulates release of pancreatic insulin	4 mg prior to meal	Short-acting!	Don't take if skipping meal	Titrate to meals	0.5–2.0
Metformin (biguanide)	Decreases hepatic glucose production, increase peripheral insulin sensitivity	Start 500–800 mg qd, max 850 mg tid	Lactic acidosis, diarrhea, nausea	Cr > 1.4, liver disease, alcohol abuse, CHF, acute illness	Periodic Cr/CBC	1.5–2.0
Glipizide sulfonylurea	Increases pancreatic insulin release	Start 2.5–5 mg qd; max 20 mg bid	Hypoglycemia; 90% liver excr. t1/2 12–24 hour.	Liver disease	BG daily when increasing dose	2.0
Glyburide sulfonylurea	Same as glipizide	Start 1.25–2.5 mg qd; max 20 mg qd	Hypoglycemia; mostly renal excr.; t1/2 24 hour.	Renal disease	BG daily when increasing dose	2.0
Acarbose (alpha-glucosidase inhibitor)	Delays breakdown/absorption of carbohydrates in gut	Start 25 mg tid, increase to 100 mg tid	Flatulence, abdominal pain, dose-depd. liver toxicity	GI disorders, liver disease	LFT q. three months for one year, then periodic	0.5–1.5
Rosiglitazone (and other glitazones)	Promotes muscle and fat glucose uptake	Start 4 mg qd increase to bid	Liver toxicity fluid retention	ALT > 1.5x nl.	ALT q. month for six months, then periodic	1.0–1.5

The metformin/sulfonylurea combination would be a good start in this obese patient; you could work to build both doses while managing diet/lifestyle issues. A third oral, rosiglitazone, could be attempted before insulin is introduced. A lipid-lowering agent should be started independently given similar side-effect profiles.

QUESTIONS

197. All of the following are indicated annually for patients with type 2 DM except:
    A. Dilated retinal exam by an eye care specialist and treatment of retinopathy
    B. Urine protein, if normal screen for microalbuminuria; ACE inhibitor for microalbuminuria or proteinuria
    C. Microfilament testing of feet
    D. Hemoglobin A1C measurement

198. The following vaccination schedule is indicated in diabetic patients:
    A. Yearly influenza, Pneumovax every five years
    B. Yearly influenza, one-time Pneumovax, and Td (tetanus) every five years
    C. Yearly influenza only
    D. Pneumovax one-time, yearly PPD

199. The leading cause of death in patients with diabetes is:
    A. Renal failure
    B. Cardiovascular disease
    C. Amputation complications
    D. Infection

200. Which of the following medicines is most effective and inexpensive in treating diabetic neuropathy?
    A. Gabapentin
    B. Tricyclic antidepressants
    C. Carbamazepine
    D. Mexilitine

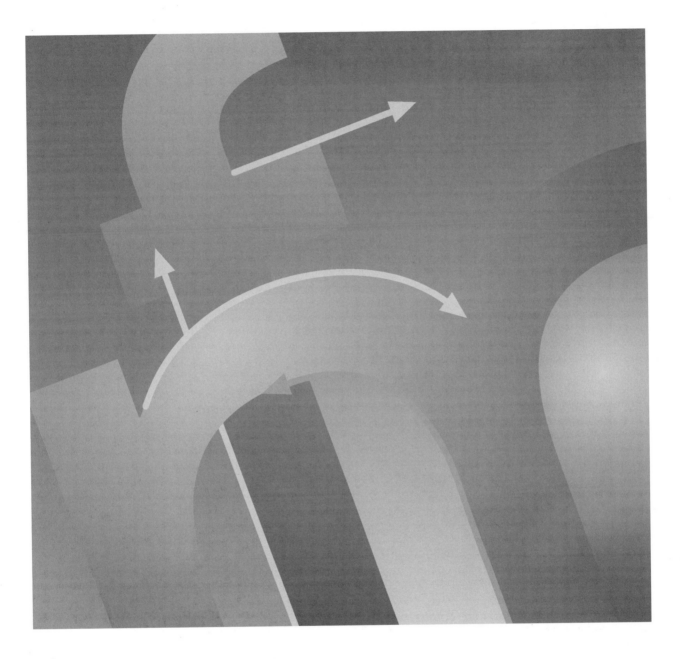

ANSWERS

CASE PRESENTATIONS

PATIENTS WHO PRESENT WITH OBSTETRIC ISSUES
Case 1. Prenatal Care
Case 2. Pregnancy and Hypertension
Case 3. First Trimester Vaginal Bleeding
Case 4. Labor

CASES THAT PRESENT IN WOMEN
Case 5. Breast Mass
Case 6. Urinary Incontinence
Case 7. Menopause
Case 8. Abnormal Pap
Case 9. Birth Control Management
Case 10. STDs

CASES THAT PRESENT IN CHILDREN
Case 11. Baby's Barking Cough
Case 12. Newborn Issues
Case 13. "My Son Has Trouble at School"
Case 14. Amenorrhea in an Adolescent
Case 15. Left Arm Pain in a 3-Year-Old Boy
Case 16. Newborn Jaundice
Case 17. School Forms

PATIENTS WHO PRESENT WITH DERMATOLOGIC ISSUES
Case 18. Skin Lesion
Case 19. Rash
Case 20. Facial Rash

PATIENTS WHO PRESENT WITH SURGICAL ISSUES
Case 21. Inguinal Mass
Case 22. Abdominal Pain

PATIENTS WHO PRESENT WITH NEUROLOGIC COMPLAINTS
Case 23. Headache
Case 24. Droopy Mouth
Case 25. Headache #2
Case 26. "I'm Dizzy"

**PATIENTS WHO PRESENT WITH CARDIOVASCULAR
OR PULMONARY COMPLAINTS**
Case 27. Chest Pain
Case 28. Short of Breath
Case 29. Chronic Cough
Case 30. Dyspnea on Exertion
Case 31. Smoker with URI

PATIENTS WHO PRESENT WITH MUSCULOSKELETAL COMPLAINTS
Case 32. Swollen Leg
Case 33. Tingling Feet
Case 34. Ankle Swelling
Case 35. Monoarticular Arthritis
Case 36. Joint Pain
Case 37. Flank Pain
Case 38. Low Back Pain

PATIENTS WHO PRESENT WITH URINARY OR GI COMPLAINTS
Case 39. Decreased Urine Output
Case 40. Bloody Diarrhea
Case 41. Hematemesis

**PATIENTS WHO PRESENT WITH PSYCHIATRIC
OR SUBSTANCE ABUSE ISSUES**
Case 42. The Shakes
Case 43. Agitation

PATIENTS WHO PRESENT WITH PRIMARY CARE ISSUES
Case 44. Obesity
Case 45. Colon Cancer Screening
Case 46. Trisomy 21
Case 47. Checkup
Case 48. Feeling Fifty
Case 49. Low Energy
Case 50. "I Can't Take My Medicines"

DIAGNOSIS

Initial OB visit
Preeclampsia
Threatened Abortion
Induction

Fibrocystic Breast Disease
Stress Incontinence
HRT, Osteoporosis
CIN 1, HPV
OCPs, Depo-Provera
Pelvic Inflammatory Disease

Pediatrics Respiratory ID; Croup
Circumcision, Breastfeeding
Attention Deficit Hyperactivity Disorder
Anorexia
Radial Head Subluxation/Child Abuse
Physiologic Jaundice
Immunizations

Melanoma
Tinea Corporis
Rosacea, Seborrheic Dermatitis

Inguinal Hernia
Cholecystitis, R/O Appendicitis

Cluster Headache
Bell's Palsy
Hypertensive Emergency
Neurocardiogenic Syncope

Coronary Artery Disease/Angina
COPD/Asthma
Tuberculosis Issues
Atrial Fibrillation
Smoking Cessation, Depression

Deep Venous Thrombosis
Macrocytic Anemia—Pernicious Anemia
Congestive Heart Failure
Gout
Osteoarthritis
Pyelonephritis/Nephrolithiasis
Prostate Cancer

Acute Renal Failure
Inflammatory Bowel Disease
Upper GI Bleed/Liver Cirrhosis/Hepatic Encephalopathy

Alcohol Withdrawal Syndrome
Delirium in Geriatric Patient

Size-Positive Approach to Weight Management
Evidence-Based Medicine Basics
Obstructive Sleep Apnea
Microcytic Anemia—Thalassemia
Hyperlipidemia
Hypothyroidism
Primary Care of Type 2 Diabetes Mellitus

1–C

Maternal tobacco use has been identified in 19–30% of pregnancies and is clearly linked with adverse pregnancy outcomes. In the United States it is responsible for approximately 20–30% of low birth weight babies and 10% of infant deaths. Smoking is also associated with an increased risk for miscarriage, abruption, placenta previa, preterm birth, and SIDS. Some of those risks (LBW, abruption) are dose-related, so encouraging a patient to smoke less each day is important if she cannot give up completely.

2–B

Gestational diabetes is the most common medical complication of pregnancy, affecting 3–6% of pregnancies in the United States. Routine screening is conducted between 24 and 28 weeks gestational age with a one-hour glucola. An abnormal value is above 140 and requires the patient to undergo a three-hour glucose tolerance test (GTT). If two or more values are abnormal on the three-hour test then the diagnosis of GDM is made. There is a "15% rule": about 15% of women will have an abnormal glucola, about 15% of those will have an abnormal three-hour GTT with a diagnosis of GDM, and about 15% of women with GDM will require insulin during their pregnancy. GDM is associated with a 50% chance of developing type II diabetes mellitus within 20 years. Of note, some authors support the use of a 135 threshold, which would increase the sensitivity, but decrease the specificity of this screening test.

3–D

The triple screen is drawn between 15 and 20 weeks gestational age and consists of maternal serum levels of AFP, hCG, and estriol.

1. An increased AFP is primarily associated with NTDs (neural tube defects), underestimated GA, multiple gestation, RH isoimmunization, and ventral wall defects.
2. A decreased AFP is associated with aneuploidy, particularly trisomy 21 and trisomy 18.
3. Adding hCG and estriol to the AFP screen can increase the sensitivity and specificity in the prenatal detection of trisomy 21, in which hCG is elevated and estriol is decreased.
4. A low value of all three tests is associated with trisomy 18.

4–B

The incidence of NTD is 1–3/1000 births. Folic acid confers a 72% protective effect against neural tube defects. The CDC recommends that all women of childbearing age who are capable of becoming pregnant should consume 0.4 mg folic acid a day. For women with a previous history of a child with NTD the recommendation is that she take 4 mg folic acid/day from four weeks before conception until 12 weeks GA.

5–C

Criteria for severe preeclampsia include SBP ≥ 160, DBP ≥ 110, proteinuria > 5 gm/24 hours, oliguria < 500 cc/24 hours, increasing creatinine, persistent headache or visual symptoms, epigastric or RUQ pain, pulmonary edema, IUGR, oligohydramnios, or HELLP syndrome (hemolysis, elevated liver enzymes, low platelets). Patients with severe preeclampsia should be considered for delivery.

6–D

Preeclampsia has severe complications including HELLP, stroke, intracranial hemorrhage, hepatic rupture, abruption, eclampsia, IUGR, pulmonary edema, acute renal failure, and fetal demise. Although HELLP and subsequent DIC can result in anemia through acute blood loss and hemolysis, most preeclamptics have an elevated hematocrit because of hemoconcentration secondary to third spacing.

7–B

Standard of care is to give magnesium to a preeclamptic patient in labor for seizure prophylaxis. If her blood pressure is consistently >160/105 she can be concurrently treated with labetalol or hydralazine. Patients with preeclampsia need very careful fluid maintenance as they are at increased risk for pulmonary edema if given excessive IVF in an effort to combat their hemoconcentrated status.

8–A

Options for blood pressure control during pregnancy include methyldopa, β-blockers, or a calcium channel blocker such as nifedipine. Traditionally, many patients are placed on methyldopa; however, this medication may not be as efficacious as β-blockers or CCBs (calcium channel blockers). There are retrospective studies that associate the use of β-blockers with IUGR; however, in these nonrandomized studies it is thought that bias from the patients with worse baseline disease is actually the etiology for decrease in birth weight rather than the medication itself.

ANSWERS

ACEIs (angiotensin converting enzyme inhibitors) and ARBs (angiotensin receptor blockers) are contraindicated because of possible fetal effects. Patients with chronic hypertension are at increased risk for preterm labor (34%), IUGR (15%), preeclampsia, abruption, and stroke.

9–B

If the βhCG is greater than 1500 mIU/ml and the pregnancy is intrauterine, a gestational sac should be visualized by TVUS. By TAUS (transabdominal ultrasound) the gestational sac may not be identified until βhCG reaches 6000 mIU/ml. If βhCG is greater than these levels but the gestational sac cannot be visualized, an ectopic location should be assumed.

10–B

βhCG first appears in maternal serum seven to nine days after conception and reaches 50–250 mIU/ml by the first missed period. In an IUP the normal doubling time for βhCG is 48 to 60 hours; however, one third of ectopic pregnancies can initially have a normal doubling time. Conversely, threatened or incomplete abortions usually have abnormal doubling times. Some centers use the serum progesterone level to help diagnose ectopics; a one-time level <5 ng/ml excludes a viable pregnancy with 100% sensitivity, levels >25 ng/ml exclude ectopic pregnancy with 98% sensitivity. There is no need to correlate progesterone and βhCG levels, although at times this can be helpful.

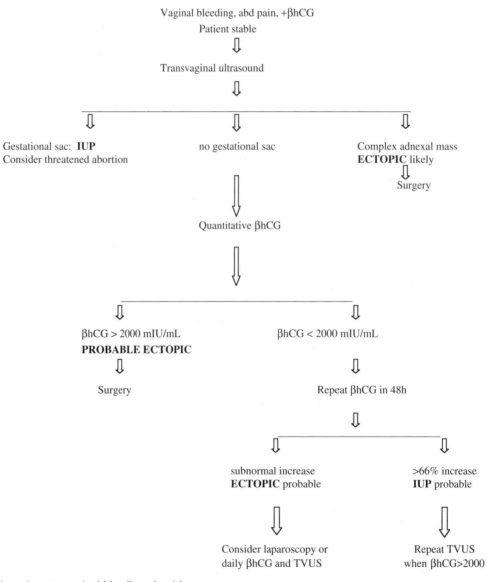

FIGURE A10 First trimester vaginal bleeding algorithm.

11–A

Ectopic pregnancies should be diagnosed and treated before the onset of hypotension and overt rupture. Surgical excision is the most common treatment modality, either by laparotomy (surgical incision into the abdomen for diagnosis and treatment) or by laparoscopy (intra-abdominal examination and treatment using an illuminated camera passed through a much smaller incision in the abdomen). Laparoscopic surgery facilitates rapid recovery, attempts to preserve fertility, and is less expensive. This is also true for medical treatment. The agent used is the folinic acid antagonist methotrexate, which inhibits synthesis of purines and pyrimidines and thus interferes with DNA synthesis and cell multiplication. Hemodynamically stable patients with ectopic pregnancies are eligible for treatment with methotrexate if the mass is unruptured and measures 4 cm or less on ultrasound. 94% of women treated with methotrexate need no further therapy.

12–A

The definitions are as follows:

TABLE A12. Types of Abortions

TYPE OF ABORTION	CERVICAL OS	TISSUE PASSED	UTERUS
Threatened	closed	no	enlarged
Inevitable	open	no	enlarged
Incomplete	open	yes	enlarged
Completed	closed	yes	small
Missed	closed	no	enlarged

(A missed abortion is different from a threatened abortion because a missed abortion is a *nonviable* pregnancy that is not yet in the process of aborting.)

13–D

Risks of Pitocin include uterine hyperstimulation, uterine rupture, and vasopressin-like effects with antidiuretic action, which can result in hyponatremia, seizures, and coma.

14–D

One of the most common side effects of epidural analgesia is maternal hypotension (≅10%). Before initiation of epidural analgesia the patient should receive prophylactic intravascular volume expansion and IV fluids. Other more serious side effects include local anesthetic toxicity (0.04%), high spinal (0.03%—anesthetic travels far enough cranially to affect the thoracic and cervical nerves and thereby suppress respirations), spinal headache (1–3%), urinary retention, epidural hematoma, or epidural abscess formation.

Studies are conflicting about the effect of epidural analgesia on labor, and many have found no mal effects. Some studies have found increased rates of instrumental vaginal deliveries; however, the majority of studies have found no increased incidence of operative or cesarean deliveries and no prolongation of labor. Therefore the standard of care is to assume that epidurals have no effect on the length of labor or the risk for cesarean section or forceps delivery.

15–D

See "Thought Question" answer in text. The patient progressed from 2 cm to 5 cm in two hours on Pitocin, received an epidural, and is having good progress. Amniotomy will help labor continue smoothly without arrest.

16–B

FHR decelerations can be classified as early, variable, and late.

Early: mirror image of contraction, secondary to head compression
Variable: herald onset of second stage of labor, secondary to umbilical cord compression, sharp in contour, need to be interpreted in light of depth, persistence, FHR variability (mild, moderate, severe)
Late: begin, peak, *and* end after contraction, significance is unrelated to the depth of the deceleration, highly suggestive of fetal acidemia if repetitive

A crash c-section would be appropriate for a severe prolonged fetal bradycardia. An urgent c-section is indicated for repetitive late decelerations.

17–D

Breast cancer lumps are often described as irregularly shaped, firm, and painless nodules, which can be fixed to the skin or muscle and are unilateral. Later findings can include erythema, edema, and retraction of the skin or nipple. Fibroadenomas are smooth and rubbery and most common in women in their 20s to 30s. Cysts are smooth-walled and somewhat tender, and occur most commonly in premenopausal women over age 40; they account for only 10% of breast masses in women under the age of 40. They tend to fluctuate with the menstrual cycle.

18–C

It can be difficult to differentiate a cyst from a solid mass on physical exam, and an ultrasound

ANSWERS

or aspiration is necessary for definitive diagnosis. After aspiration, a surgical biopsy is indicated only if the fluid is bloody, if the mass doesn't resolve completely after aspiration, or if the same cyst recurs multiple times. Otherwise, the patient can simply be re-examined in four to six weeks to document that the cyst has not recurred and that no other masses are palpable.

19–A

A solid mass requires histologic diagnosis, either by fine needle aspiration biopsy, by core needle biopsy, or by excisional biopsy. Fine needle aspiration uses a 20-Ga. needle to obtain samples from the mass for cytology and is around 90% sensitive and 98% specific. A core needle biopsy uses a 14-Ga. needle to remove cores, and requires a small skin incision and local anesthesia. An excisional biopsy is done when a needle biopsy is negative but the mass is clinically suspicious for cancer, and may even be the procedure of choice if the probability of malignancy is high based on the H&P. An ultrasound or mammogram is also useful to document the extent of the mass and rule out the presence of other lesions. However, in the presence of a breast mass a normal mammogram should never be considered proof of absence of breast cancer as 9–22% of palpable breast cancers are not seen on mammogram.

20–D

Although there is some variation between different task force recommendations, routine breast cancer screening should include yearly clinical breast exam and annual mammograms starting at age 50. It has been firmly established in several RCTs (randomized controlled trials) that periodic mammograms in asymptomatic women ages 50–75 will decrease breast cancer mortality by 20–30%. Although mammographic screening of women ages 40 to 49 remains controversial, recent studies seem to indicate reduction in breast cancer mortality in this age group as well. Clinical breast exams have also been shown to reduce mortality, and in some studies have the same sensitivity on their own as clinical breast exam plus mammography. Although many physicians teach patients how to do a self breast exam (SBE), limited data exist to quantify the value of SBE. Recent studies have provided conflicting results on the efficacy of this intervention, and for now performing SBE is best left up to the patient after informed discussion with her physician.

21–D

Stress incontinence is due to a combination of 1) urethral hypermobility (secondary to loss of support at the urethrovesical junction) and 2) intrinsic urethral sphincter deficiency (bladder neck is open at rest, which often occurs in older women, hypoestrogenic states, after trauma, pelvic surgery, radiation therapy, or certain neurological lesions).

Labor and vaginal delivery can damage the pelvic floor. Increased intra-abdominal pressure from chronic coughing or constipation is also a risk factor, and as with all forms of neuromuscular injury, aging seems to worsen the problem.

22–A

Kegel exercises are pelvic muscle exercises which decrease the episodes of incontinence by 40–60% in clinical trials. In fact, in some very teaching-intensive trials success rates rose as high as a 95% reduction of incontinence episodes. Along with Kegel exercises, newly diagnosed patients should be told to avoid liquids after dinner, decline caffeinated beverages, empty their bladders around the clock, and keep a voiding/intake diary.

Medications can be an important adjunct therapy for many patients.

- Urge incontinence responds best to anticholinergic medications, which relax the detrusor muscle and decrease spasms; a popular choice is tolterodine or oxybutynin.
- Stress incontinence can be treated with hormone replacement therapy, either topically or orally, to strengthen the vaginal tissues and amplify periurethral blood flow. Alpha-agonists such as pseudoephedrine increase the muscle tone of the urethral sphincter, bladder base, and bladder neck, creating a stronger seal against leakage.
- Mixed incontinence responds well to imipramine, a combined alpha-agonist and anticholinergic medication.

Surgery is helpful for SI patients who have not responded to other modalities; which surgery is done depends on the exact anatomical etiology of the incontinence. Bladder neck suspension results in an 80% cure rate, anterior vaginal repair gives a 65% cure, sling procedures and periurethral bulking injections are quoted as having an 80–90% cure rate.

23–D

Patients to refer for further urodynamic testing and evaluation by a specialist include those with a history of previous pelvic surgery, patients with hematuria without infection on urinalysis, patients with gross pelvic prolapse, or patients with an abnormal post-void residual.

24–A

Patients who suffer from both detrusor instability and genuine stress incontinence are said to have mixed incontinence. The important point here is that patients usually cannot distinguish between the two, and because of the high prevalence of mixed incontinence, it is important to include simple or complex urodynamic studies in the evaluation. Although medications such as imipramine treat both kinds of incontinence, most other medical and surgical treatments only target one kind of incontinence.

25–D

The only absolute contraindications to HRT include active liver disease, unexplained vaginal bleeding, active thromboembolic disease, uncontrolled hypertension, porphyria, and a personal history of an estrogen-dependent cancer (breast, uterine). Some relative contraindications include symptomatic gallbladder disease, pancreatitis, marked hypertriglyceridemia, and migraines exacerbated by estrogen.

26–C

Alternatives to hormones do exist and some large studies have shown modest improvement for some remedies, however none as effective as HRT. Such alternatives include:

Vasomotor and GU symptoms: clonidine, vitamin E, vaginal lubricants, phytoestrogens (soy, oats, buckwheat, barley, corn), belladonna
Hyperlipidemia: exercise, weight loss, improved eating habits, raloxifene
Osteoporosis: calcium, vitamin D, raloxifene, exercise, calcitonin, alendronate, bisphosphonates

Alternatives that are very popular among patients but have shown no benefit in studies include black cohosh, dong quai, evening primrose, St. John's wort, koo sar, and wild yam creams.

27–B

More than 40% of women have fractures by the age of 80, and more than 70% after age 80. Risk factors include female gender, family history of osteoporosis, Caucasian or Asian race, nulliparous women, lack of exercise, poor calcium intake,

smoking, history of steroid use, high caffeine or alcohol intake, thyroid disease, and use of anticonvulsants. Women with any risk factors at all should be screened with a DXA (dual x-ray photon absorptiometry) scan to measure the central bone mineral density. The results are reported as a T-score (the number of standard deviations the patient's BMD [bone mineral density] varies from the mean of young adult women) and a Z-score (the number of standard deviations the patient's BMD varies from age/sex/race-matched controls). According to World Health Organization standards, osteoporosis is present when the T-score is at least 2.5 standard deviations below the norm.

The WHO definition is based on the T-score, and in general few practicing physicians use the Z-score to aid with diagnosis or treatment decisions. The T-score is based on the BMD of young adult women because this is considered to be the *peak* of bone mass; for each SD below peak bone mass (or one-unit decrease in T-score) a woman's fracture risk doubles.

28–A

Although the patient has few risk factors for endometrial cancer, any postmenopausal patient with unexplained vaginal bleeding needs a workup to exclude endometrial cancer. 90% of women with endometrial cancer present with vaginal bleeding; however, you must also be sure to tell the patient that most vaginal bleeding is not cancer. Risk factors for endometrial cancer include age over 55, obesity, nulliparous, diabetes, hypertension, liver disease, early menarche, hirsutism, and a history of taking unopposed estrogen. The workup includes an endometrial biopsy done easily in the office, a Pap smear and exam to exclude a cervical source for the bleeding, and a pelvic ultrasound. An endometrial stripe greater than 5 mm wide on ultrasound is suspicious. Definitive diagnosis can be made with a D&C in the OR.

29–B

Although the CIN I is likely to regress and the patient could elect to proceed without treatment and careful follow-up with Paps, the patient would like treatment. Cryotherapy is easy, is inexpensive, and has a low complication rate. It is best for small lesions that are mildly or moderately dysplastic. LEEP is also an office procedure, takes a little more skill to perform, and can accommodate larger lesions. Both LEEP and cryotherapy are considered *ablative* therapies and require that

ANSWERS

the colposcopy was satisfactory, that the ECC was negative, and that the whole lesion can be seen.

A cone biopsy is indicated when the criteria for ablative therapy are not met. Conization is both a diagnostic and therapeutic procedure and has the advantage over ablative therapy of providing tissue for further pathologic evaluation to rule out invasive cancer.

30–B

Immunosuppression can accelerate cervical dysplastic changes. In HIV-positive women *any* abnormal Pap smear at all requires immediate colposcopy because of the rapidity of progression to invasive cancer.

31–A

Data have firmly established that HPV DNA are detected in most women with cervical neoplasia. The percentage of CIN apparently attributable to HPV approaches 90%. Although the number of known genital HPV types now exceeds 20, only certain types are "high-risk" and count for approximately 90% of HGSIL and cancer. Type 16 is the most common HPV type in invasive cancer, CIN II, and CIN III, and is found in 47% of women.

Most HPV infections do not persist. Most women have no apparent clinical evidence of disease and the infection is eventually suppressed or eliminated spontaneously. A minority of women exposed to HPV develops persistent infection that can progress to CIN; factors that may have a role in this progression include smoking, infection with other STDs, immune suppression, and poor nutrition.

32–B

After cryotherapy the patient will have a heavy discharge for several weeks. After three months the cervix has had a chance to heal and a Pap smear is important to document eradication of the abnormal cells. Once the patient has a normal post-treatment Pap smear she can continue with the ACOG (American College of Obstetrics and Gynecology) screening recommendations for annual Pap and pelvic exams. The recommendations state that after a woman has three or more normal Paps, the Pap smear can be performed "at the discretion of her physician."

33–B

Noncontraceptive benefits of OCPs include a reduced incidence of PID, less acne, less hirsutism, increased bone density, decreased menstrual blood loss, decreased incidence of ectopic pregnancy, less dysmenorrhea, less benign breast disease, and a decreased incidence of endometrial cancer and ovarian cancer.

Side effects of OCPs can include nausea, two to five pound weight gain with the higher-dose pills, spotting in between menses, headache, mood swings, and occasionally amenorrhea.

34–B

Although all the options would be important to review, in this 17-year-old healthy patient the only contraindication of the four would be a history of DVT and possible hypercoagulability. In general, contraindications to OCPs include thrombotic disease, history of CVA or CAD, breast cancer, liver tumor, impaired liver function, smoker older than age 35, SLE, active gallbladder disease, and undiagnosed vaginal bleeding. Relative contraindications include migraines, hypertension, and concurrent anticonvulsants (unless on the progestin-only pills).

The DVT risk for women on OCPs is 10–30/100,000 vs. 60/100,000 in pregnant women and 4/100,000 in non-OCP users.

35–D

8% of women having sex during the second to third week of their cycle get pregnant; 12–30% get pregnant if they have sex in the one to two days around ovulation. Requirements for emergency contraception include a history of unprotected intercourse in the past 72 hours and a negative pregnancy test. Contraindications to emergency contraception include recent CVA or MI, active liver disease, active thromboembolic disease, pregnancy, or breast or endometrial cancer. Emergency contraception pills are estimated to reduce the risk of pregnancy by 75%.

36–D

Depo-Provera side effects include irregular bleeding initially with most patients being amenorrheic after the second shot, decreased bone density, headache, and dizziness.

37–D

The most common complication of gonorrhea in women is PID, which occurs in 10–20% of infected women. Other complications include Bartholin's abscess, perihepatitis, conjunctivitis, disseminated gonococcal infection, septic abortion, preterm labor, and infertility.

A wet mount involves placing a drop of saline on a slide which has already been smeared with the discharge using a Q-tip. Bacterial vaginosis can be diagnosed with *clue cells*, vaginal squamous cells with the edges studded with bacteria. If you look quickly after doing the pelvic exam, trichomonads can be seen swimming in the saline using their flagella. Another slide with the discharge is mixed with a drop of KOH, used to lyse the cell walls and therefore distinguish the hypha of a fungal infection more easily.

The patient's negative wet mount makes *Trichomonas* or bacterial vaginosis unlikely causes of her vaginal discharge. The negative KOH prep makes a candidal etiology less likely.

38-A

PID usually results from the ascending spread of microorganisms from the vagina and endocervix to the upper genital tract. Each year 1 million women in the United States are diagnosed with PID; between 10% and 40% of women with untreated gonococcal or chlamydial cervicitis will develop PID. Laparoscopy is considered the gold standard diagnosis, however is not feasible or appropriate in the majority of cases. Therefore, PID is a clinical diagnosis based on the following minimum criteria in the absence of a competing diagnosis: lower abdominal tenderness, bilateral adnexal tenderness, and cervical motion tenderness. Additional criteria to consider include fever, abnormal discharge, elevated ESR, and laboratory evidence of infection with *N. gonorrhea* or *C. trachomatis*. All women should have a pregnancy test, and women with severe pain should have an ultrasound to exclude a TOA.

39-A

Criteria for hospitalization for treatment of PID include pregnancy, inability to exclude a surgical emergency (appendicitis, etc.), poor clinical response to oral outpatient antimicrobial therapy, inability to tolerate or follow an outpatient oral regimen, severe illness, fever, nausea, or vomiting, TOA, and immunodeficiency.

Inpatient Meds:
1) cefotetan or ceftriaxone + doxycycline
2) clindamycin + gentamycin + doxycycline
3) ciprofloxacin + doxycycline + metronidazole
4) ofloxacin + metronidazole
5) ampicillin/sulbactam + doxycycline

Outpatient Meds:
1) ceftriaxone or cefoxitin IM + doxycycline
2) ofloxacin + metronidazole

40–B

Common sequelae of PID include infertility, chronic pelvic pain, and ectopic pregnancy. The risk for ectopic pregnancy rises sevenfold after a single episode of PID and 12% of women are infertile. After two episodes of PID 25% of women are infertile, and after three episodes 50% are. Many women exhibit mild or subtle symptoms and are not diagnosed with PID; many women with infertility have no known history of the disease.

41–B

Clinicians can be guided by the clinical croup score below in assessing the severity of airway obstruction.

TABLE A41. Clinical Croup Scores			
	0	1	2
insp. breath sounds	normal	harsh with rhonchi	delayed
stridor at rest	none	inspiratory	inspiratory/ expiratory
cough	none	hoarse cry	bark
retractions/ flaring	none	flaring and suprasternal retractions	at left +sub- and intercostal retractions
cyanosis	none	in air	in 40% O_2

A score of 4 indicates moderate croup, >7 necessitates ICU admission. Our patient has at maximum a score of 3 and is clinically well hydrated. Because he is relatively early in the time-course of the disease, follow-up in 24 hours is warranted. Racemic epinephrine given with or without IM steroids can help moderate the course of the disease, but you need to have time to observe the child after the treatment has worn off in two hours. Humidified oxygen can help the moderately stridorous child, but lateral neck radiographs would not assist the clinical diagnosis in this patient.

42–A

The "steeple sign," narrowing of the laryngeal air column below the vocal cords, was once thought to be pathognomonic for viral laryngotracheitis. However, it may be absent in some children with clinical croup and present as a normal variant in others. It is not necessary for the diagnosis of croup. Flattened diaphragms are seen in hypeinflation, such as with asthma. A deviated trachea can be seen with pneumothorax or pulmonary mass. Fluffy infiltrates would be more consistent with atypical pneumonia.

ANSWERS

43–D

Bacterial tracheitis (membranous tracheitis) is a fulminant bacterial infection that can quickly proceed to full airway obstruction. Pus may be expelled during the barking cough. It necessitates rapid intubation and aggressive antibiotic therapy.

44–D

Chronic stridor in a young infant is most often due to a congenital anomaly like laryngomalacia or tracheoesophageal fistula.

45–C

Almost all uncircumcised boys will have tight foreskins for the first year. 50% of 2-year-olds will have fully retractable foreskins, as will 90% of 3-year-olds. In some normal boys, it will not fully retract until school age. It is most important never to forcibly retract the foreskin, as this will lyse the protective adhesions between the glans and the foreskin and may lead to phimosis or infection. When the foreskin naturally retracts, penile hygiene can be performed at bath time.

46–D

Circumcised babies do feel pain and have the right to analgesia during the procedure. A dorsal penile nerve block (with xylocaine, no epinephrine) is more effective than topical cream, decreasing crying time and heart rate response, but lidocaine-prilocaine cream is also effective. Dorsal penile nerve block does not cause penile necrosis. Untreated circumcision pain has been linked not only to short-term alterations in crying, but also to increased pain with vaccinations through 6 months of age.

47–A

Cow's milk and some formulas contain mostly casein; breast milk contains mostly whey. Whey is less allergenic than casein in the first 6 months of age. White blood cells and immunoglobulins are an important component in breast milk and not only protect from and fight infection but also help seal the gut to prevent allergy formation. Cholesterol may help induce cholesterol metabolism in the liver and is also a source of components for myelin.

48–C

Preterm infants may benefit greatly from breast milk, for all of the reasons listed above. A fortifier may be needed for certain preterm infants. All of the listed infections, as well as active substance abuse in the mother, are contraindications for breastfeeding. HIV is passed through breast milk, and is an absolute contraindication regardless of treatment status.

49–A

Decreased appetite is found in up to 80% of children taking methylphenidate; 10–15% have significant weight loss. Insomnia is reported in 3%–85%, and tachycardia is more pronounced at rest. These drugs may slow weight gain and growth slightly, but there has been no documented attributable height loss. Pemoline can cause toxic hepatitis. Transient tics may be provoked, which usually decrease over time.

50–B

ADHD affects boys two to five times more than girls. If applied to a prevalence of ADHD of 10%, that would mean that up to one in six boys would have ADHD. The prevalence of ADHD has been estimated between 1.7% and 17.8% of the population—clearly the interpretation of the DSM-IV criteria varies widely.

51–C

In addition to oppositional defiant disorder, alcoholism, conduct disorder, and learning disabilities, depression and anxiety disorders are also common.

52–C

Symptoms of ADHD usually lessen over time, but up to 50% of patients carry the diagnosis to adulthood. ADHD children do well socially in a regular classroom, possibly with modifications to the classroom and teaching method.

53–D

Vitiligo is not a physical manifestation of anorexia nervosa; it is a dermatologic condition characterized by depigmented plaques. Signs of the eating disorder include temporal wasting, hypothermia, lanugo hair over the body, bradycardia, cardiac failure, malnutrition, infertility secondary to amenorrhea, anemia, and depression or anxiety. Osteoporosis is often overlooked, and can be a serious complication.

54–C

The leading causes of death in adolescents are motor vehicle accidents, homicides, suicides, then all other causes. It is important, therefore, to ask adolescents about these areas in order to risk-stratify and determine appropriate interventions.

55–C

Hemoglobin A1C is a test correlating with long-term hyperglycemia in the management of a patient with diabetes mellitus; it would not be useful in a patient with anorexia nervosa. No single laboratory test is diagnostic for anorexia, as the diagnosis is a clinical one. Certain tests should be obtained, however, to determine any complications from the disease that can be treated. A CBC, basic metabolic panel, liver function tests, calcium, magnesium, phosphate, and thyroid function tests should be ordered initially. If amenorrhea persists for a prolonged length of time, bone densitometry should be ordered, given the patient's high risk for osteoporosis and complicating fractures.

56–D

All of the questions listed should be asked of an adolescent patient. After ensuring confidentiality with an adolescent patient while talking with him or her alone, the important topics to discuss are those in which adolescents are most at risk. A good mnemonic to remember is HEADS. This captures important areas to discuss with an adolescent.

Home—ask about the patient's life at home, who lives with him or her, how those relationships are, what the family life is like

Education—ask about school, friends, grade-level, grades, subjects

Activities—ask about extracurricular activities, hobbies, what he or she likes to do in free time, with whom he or she spends time

Abuse—ask about abuse, sexual or physical, and any violence the patient may encounter

Drugs—ask about drug use, including tobacco, alcohol, marijuana; if any positive answers, should continue the drug screen to include other substances

Depression—ask about mood states

Sex—ask about sexual relationships, partners, STDs, use of condoms and contraception

Suicide—ask about suicidal thoughts or attempts, especially if any noted depression

57–C

A transverse long-bone fracture in a 10-year-old is a plausible injury for age, and would not be suspicious for abuse. Fractures that have high specificity for abuse are metaphysial fractures, posterior rib fractures, scapular fractures, spinous process fractures, and sternal fractures.

58–A

The law requires that any *suspected* cases of child abuse be reported. If a physician appropriately reports a suspected case, he or she is protected from any lawsuits. The term "child abuse" is a legal term, not a medical diagnosis. Documentation of injuries or findings in any suspected case of abuse should be clear, detailed, descriptive, without judgment as to cause of the finding or lack of finding. Photographs are essential.

59–D

Neglect has the greatest reported incidence, 54%; followed by physical abuse, 25%; sexual abuse, 11%; emotional abuse, 3%. It is important to remember, however, that there is much underreporting of all types of abuse, especially those without physical evidence (neglect and emotional abuse).

60–A

Child abuse is 15 times more likely to occur in families with spousal violence. Most abuse takes place in the home environment by a known and trusted individual to the child. There is no difference in the incidence of child abuse in rural and urban settings.

61–A

Physiologic jaundice is indirect; the direct component is <2 mg/dl. Schistocytes on a peripheral blood smear indicate hemolysis. A cephalohematoma would cause an indirect bilirubinemia, but is not defined as physiologic jaundice (non-pathologic). An indirect bilirubin level of 20 mg/dl should be closely monitored and, depending on etiology, should be treated with phototherapy and/or exchange transfusions. This high level would not be consistent with physiologic jaundice, which usually peaks at levels of 13–15 mg/dl.

62–D

A positive Babinski response (toe extension in response to plantar stimulation; "upgoing toes") can be elicited in some normal infants until 2 years of age, after which it becomes an abnormal reflex. The Moro response (startle reflex) should disappear by 6 months; persistence indicates neurologic disease. The palmar reflex (grasping reflex) disappears by 3 to 4 months; persistence indicates CNS dysfunction. The trunk incurvation (Galant's)

ANSWERS

reflex (stroking the back 1 cm lateral to the spine invokes curving of the trunk to the stimulated side) disappears at 2 months; an absent reflex at birth indicates spinal cord lesions.

63–D

Biliary atresia causes a direct (conjugated) hyper-bilirubinemia. The hepatocytes can conjugate and process bilirubin, but obstruction prevents further metabolism, leading to increased serum levels of direct bilirubin. Delayed clamping of the cord at delivery can cause polycythemia in the infant, and breakdown of the increased load of RBCs will ulti-mately yield increased indirect (unconjugated) hyperbilirubinemia. Likewise, a cephalohematoma, or other significant bruising, causes increased RBC breakdown and indirect bilirubin. Isoimmunization (via Rh or other antibodies) causes hemolysis and increased indirect bilirubin.

64–B

Kernicterus is caused by bilirubin staining of the basal ganglia and hippocampus. The neurologic sequelae include hypotonia, lethargy, seizures, hearing loss, and mental retardation.

65–C

Inactivated poliovirus is recommended for all polio vaccinations because the oral poliovirus has an increased risk of vaccine-associated paralytic poliomyelitis.

66–A

The MMR vaccine is formed of attenuated live virus. It should not be given to pregnant women because the rubella component induces the risk of teratogenicity (congenital rubella syndrome, characterized by microcephaly, mental retarda-tion, and deafness). Allergies to eggs and neomycin are absolute contraindications to immunization with MMR.

67–D

Hepatitis B vaccine is a genetically engineered antigen, yeast recombinant antigen. Other vac-cines are: tetanus—bacterial toxoid; pertussis—killed whole organism bacteria; Hib—bacterial conjugate; MMR—live attenuated virus.

68–B

The categories of development screened by the Denver II are personal-social, fine motor-adaptive, language, and gross motor.

69–C

It is imperative that all suspicious pigmented lesions be biopsied to rule out malignant melanoma. This patient has several risk factors for melanoma (Caucasian, chronic sun exposure, family history, enlarging lesion in a sun-exposed area, lesion bleeds) and the lesion fits the ABCDE criteria (asymmetry, border irregularity, color variegation, diameter more than 6 mm, elevation). An increase in size or a change in color of the lesion is noted in at least 70% of patients who have melanoma.

70–C

TABLE A70. Biopsy Types		
	PROS	CONS
Shave biopsy	quick	potential bisection of melanoma false neg when pathology is in deeper
Excisional biopsy	improved sensitivity evaluation of deeper path	increased time for procedure large skin defect
Punch biopsy	rapid, safe, simple useful for multiple biopsies	may be inadequate for deep path can cause scarring if large
Incisional biopsy	diagnosis of large lesions	scarring, bleeding

71–B

Basal cell carcinoma comprises 60% of all primary skin cancers, but is so slow-growing that it rarely metastasizes. Squamous cell carcinoma makes up 20% of all cases of skin cancer, and typically occurs on sun-exposed areas, areas that have been sub-jected to ionizing radiation, or areas that involved chronic inflammation or irritation. Malignant melanoma comprises only 1% of skin cancers, but accounts for greater than 60% of skin cancer deaths. The occurrence of melanoma has risen rap-idly over the past several decades, with the life-time risk now approaching 1/100. Melanoma represents 1% of all cancer deaths in the U.S. Kaposi's sarcoma is a vascular tumor that occurs most commonly in patients with immune deficien-cies and elderly patients of Mediterranean origin.

72–B

Electrodessication and curettage is best for nodu-lar basal cell cancers less than 6 mm in diameter and small squamous cell cancers. Larger tumors or those near the vermilion border of the lip are best excised. Radiation is helpful for elderly patients who cannot tolerate even minor surgical procedures. Tumors in cosmetically sensitive areas can be beautifully treated with Mohs' micrographic surgery. 5-FU can target very superficial SCC or BCC. Best options:

BCC: surgical excision, E&C, XRT
SCC: surgical excision, XRT
MM: surgical excision with wide margin

73–A

The history and physical is classic for a superficial fungal infection. These infections are caused by dermatophytes, yeasts, and molds. It is estimated that 10–20% of the world's population is infected by a dermatophyte. The term "tinea" refers exclusively to dermatophyte infections; they are classified according to their anatomic location: tinea manuum (hand), tinea pedis (foot), tinea cruris (groin), tinea corporis (body), tinea capitis (scalp), tinea unguium (nail), tinea barbae (beard). Most fungal infections do not fluoresce under Wood's lamp, and KOH microscopy shows hyphae in the case of dermatophytes, and pseudohyphae or yeast forms in yeast (*Candida*) infections. If the physical exam is suspicious for a fungal infection and microscopy is positive, there is no need for a fungal culture.

Because the patient in the case used a steroid cream first, the classic clinical presentation was altered on the repeat PE two weeks later. Steroid creams suppress the inflammation that attempts to contain the fungal infection, resulting in faster growth of the rash with obliteration of the borders and appearance of red papules within the rash. This is called "tinea incognito."

74–C

Dermatophytes, specifically *Trichophyton*, *Epidermophyton*, and *Microsporum* species, are responsible for most superficial fungal infections. The most common cause of tinea corporis is *Trichophyton rubrum*. Tinea corporis is also known as "ringworm." Lesions begin as flat, scaly spots that then develop a raised border that extends out at variable rates in all directions.

75–B

As this patient has a localized lesion, topical treatment is adequate; for more generalized cases consider oral antifungals. Oral therapy is often chosen because of its shorter duration and the potential for greater patient compliance.

OTC creams: Desenex, Tinactin, clotrimazole, miconazole, terbinafine
Prescription creams: econazole, ketoconazole, butenafine

76–D

Oral antifungals include griseofulvin, ketoconazole, fluconazole, itraconazole, and terbinafine. For optimal absorption griseofulvin should be taken with a fatty meal, whereas itraconazole and ketoconazole rely on gastric acidity for optimal absorption. All patients on these medications should have a baseline CBC and LFTs, with repeat labs if therapy lasts more than six weeks. They all inhibit the cytochrome P450 enzyme system and thus interact with many common medications. Other side effects of these medications include rash, headache, and GI distress.

77–D

Rosacea is a chronic, progressive dermatosis characterized by flushing and blushing, facial erythema, papules and pustules, telangiectasia, and potential hyperplasia of the soft tissues of the face, particularly the nose. The etiology is unknown, but is somehow associated with inappropriate vasodilation of the facial vessels. The prevalence is estimated at 5–10%, and rosacea occurs mostly between the ages of 30 and 60. The most common sites are the cheeks, nose, chin, and forehead. Complications include edema of the face, rhinophyma, dry eye and blepharitis, gram-negative folliculitis, and pyoderma faciale (painful, deep-seated nodules containing large amounts of sterile purulent material).

78–D

Treatment not only controls current symptoms but also helps prevent further eruptions. Rosacea develops gradually and is exacerbated by heat, sun, cold, wind, exercise, alcohol, spicy foods, and other irritating factors such as soaps, astringents, and benzoyl peroxide. The patient should use a mild nonsoap bar and start on combination therapy with an oral and a topical antibiotic.

Oral: tetracycline
        erythromycin
        doxycycline
        minocycline
        clarithromycin
        trimethoprim/sulfamethoxazole
        ampicillin
        metronidazole
Topical: metronidazole 0.75–1%
        clindamycin
        sulfacetamide sodium 10%

ANSWERS

79–A

Although the rash may initially sound the same, the niece's age and the description of the rash suggest seborrheic dermatitis. Scaling and eczematous changes differentiate this condition from rosacea, as well as the pattern of distribution, which includes the paranasal area, nasolabial folds, and areas beyond the face.

Atopic dermatitis presents first and foremost with pruritus. The rash consists of erythema, papules, and lichenification (thickening of the epidermis) and is typically found in the flexural regions in adults.

Psoriasis is composed of very distinct lesions, which begin as red, scaling papules that coalesce to form round plaques. The scale is adherent and silvery white. Psoriasis affects the extensor surfaces and scalp, and usually spares the palms, soles, and face.

Seborrheic dermatitis affects people from birth into the 60s, and appears in areas of increased sebaceous gland activity, such as the eyebrows, nasolabial folds, scalp, ears, groin, and chest. It may be hormonally dependent, and is also associated with proliferation of the resident fungus *Pityrosporum ovale*. It is frequently a presenting sign of HIV infection and is found in up to 85% of infected persons.

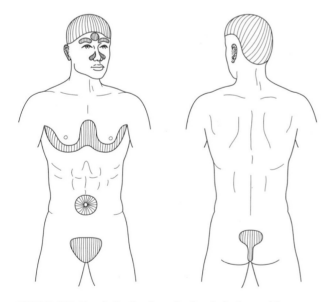

FIGURE A79 Usual distribution of seborrheic dermatitis. (Illustration by Electronic Illustrators Group.)

80–D

As opposed to rosacea, frequent and vigorous cleansing with soap removes oils from affected areas and improves seborrhea, as does sun exposure.

Pharmacologic treatment options include anti-fungals, keratolytics, steroids, and sebosuppressive agents:

Antifungals: selenium shampoo
pyrithione zinc shampoo
ketoconazole shampoo
miconazole cream
clotrimazole cream
terbinafine cream
ketoconazole cream
Keratolytics: coal tar shampoo
salicylic acid shampoo
salicylic acid hair lotion
benzoyl peroxide
Steroids: fluocinolone shampoo
hydrocortisone cream
fluocinolone cream
betamethasone cream
Sebosuppressives: isotretinoin

81–C

The most common hernia in both sexes is the indirect inguinal hernia, which accounts for 50% of all hernias in adults and is 8 to 10 times more common in men. The male:female ratio is 9:1 for inguinal hernias and 1:3 for femoral hernias. Please see the above case text for a review of the difference between direct and indirect hernias.

82–A

Because the mass is able to be pushed back into the abdominal cavity with abdominal muscle relaxation, it is reducible. An incarcerated hernia is one where you are unable to reduce the contents back into the abdominal cavity. A strangulated hernia is an incarcerated hernia in which the patient also shows signs of intestinal obstruction, such as severe pain, vomiting, distention, and obstipation. Direct inguinal hernias are the least likely to become incarcerated or strangulated; femoral hernias are the most likely to become strangulated.

83–B

Most early inguinal hernias can be diagnosed by a careful physical examination such as you have done. Sonography may be useful in diagnosing inguinal hernias in patients who report symptoms but do not have a palpable defect (sensitivity and specificity more than 90%). In the extremely rare patient with inguinal pain but no physical or sonographic evidence of inguinal herniation, CT can be used to evaluate the pelvis for the presence of a hernia.

84–B

Almost all groin hernias should be surgically repaired. Your patient today presents with a symptomatic, reducible hernia, for which the appropriate treatment is elective repair for the relief of symptoms and prevention of strangulation later on. If the hernia had been incarcerated you would have attempted gentle reduction in your office and then sent him for surgical evaluation in the next day or two. A strangulated hernia needs immediate surgical decompression and repair.

Hernia repair may be performed using general, regional (spinal/epidural), or local anesthesia. Several studies have found that with proper preoperative preparation, more than 90% of groin hernias can be repaired with local anesthetic alone. Hernia repair can be done open or laparoscopically. Recurrence is the most common long-term complication of inguinal herniorrhaphy, and is reported to be between 5% and 8% for indirect inguinal hernias.

85–D

Risk factors for gallstone formation include increasing age, obesity, rapid weight loss, multiparity, estrogens, progesterones, ceftriaxone, fibrates, Pima Indian/Latin-American/Scandinavian ethnicity, family history of gallbladder disease, female gender, TPN, high triglycerides, and a history of ileal disease (fat, female, forty, fertile).

86–A

Definitions:

Biliary colic: functional spasm of the cystic duct when obstructed by stones
Cholelithiasis: stones in the gallbladder
Acute cholecystitis: gallstones obstructing cystic duct → inflammation of GB wall
Choledocholithiasis: CBD (common bile duct) stones
Cholangitis: pus in GB, usually secondary to choledocholithiasis (Charcot triad: pain, jaundice, chills) – often *E. Coli, Klebsiella, Pseudomonas, Enterococci*

Acute cholecystitis usually presents with symptoms of local inflammation, such as RUQ pain, as well as fever, leukocytosis, and possibly elevated LFTs.

Ultrasound is more than 95% sensitive and specific for the diagnosis of gallstones greater than 2 mm in diameter. Ultrasound findings that are suggestive of acute cholecystitis include pericholecystic fluid, GB wall thickening, and a Murphy's sign. Ultrasound is 85% sensitive and 92% specific for diagnosing appendicitis, and shows an inflamed appendix measuring more than 6 mm in diameter, which is incompressible and tender with focal compression.

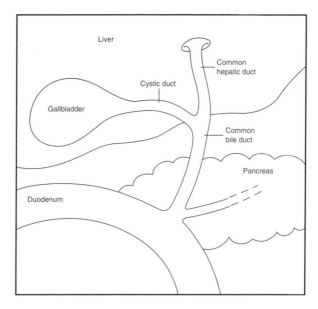

FIGURE A86 Gallbladder anatomy. (Illustration by Electronic Illustrators Group.)

87–B

Early laparoscopic cholecystectomy is indicated once the diagnosis is made and the patient is stable; it has been shown to be superior to open cholecystectomy in multiple RCTs (randomized controlled trials) with decreased postoperative pain, a shorter hospital stay, and more rapid return to work and usual activities. ERCP can be considered in patients who are at excessive risk for surgery, and is the best method for detecting choledocholithiasis (sensitivity and specificity 95%).

88–A

As many as one third of patients with gallstones will develop biliary colic and 10% develop acute cholecystitis. Other complications occur in less than 1% of cases each, and include emphysematous cholecystitis, hydrops of the gallbladder, small bowel obstruction/gallstone ileus, gastric outlet obstruction, pancreatitis, perforation of the gallbladder, and cholangitis.

ANSWERS

89–D

Migraine headache affects about 10% of adults. It is more common in women than men. The prodrome (including aura) usually lasts 15 to 30 minutes and could include visual symptoms, vertigo, aphasia, confusion, or even hemiplegia. The headache is unilateral, pulsating, intense, and may include vomiting. A prodrome or aura that persists beyond one hour may be indicative of an intracranial process such as AVM or ischemic stroke.

90–C

All of the medicines listed except progesterone are indicated, as well as calcium-channel blockers, and in refractory cases anticonvulsants. A special type of migraine, menstrual migraine, is related to the drop in estrogen prior to the initiation of menses. Oral contraceptives may mitigate the frequency and severity of migraine, but a progesterone only method would not be indicated for prophylaxis and may exacerbate migraine.

91–B

Patients with cranial or temporal arteritis often complain of scalp tenderness, especially with hair combing. The inflamed artery is not always the temporal artery, and the affected artery is not always painful or palpable. Blindness, caused by inflammation and occlusion of the ophthalmic artery, can occur one to two months after the onset of the headache and progresses quickly once visual loss starts.

92–C

Tension-type headaches are muscle contraction headaches that are highly correlated with stress, emotional strain, and depression. Chronic tension-type headaches occur 15 or more days per month. They are almost always bilateral and frequently disrupt the sleep cycle, either by inhibiting ability to fall asleep or causing early morning awakenings. Regular analgesic medication may actually cause daily headache. Tricyclic antidepressants have been shown to be beneficial, as well as relaxation and biofeedback therapy.

93–D

More than two thirds of people with Bell's palsy spontaneously and completely recover. About 15% have mild cosmetically acceptable sequelae, and another 10–15% have a permanent significant decrease in function. 85% of patients see the first signs of improvement within three weeks of onset.

94–E

The medical treatment of Bell's palsy has been greatly studied and debated. The cause of Bell's palsy is unclear; theories include autoimmune process, postviral effect, hereditary factors, and vascular ischemia. Herpes-simplex virus-1 has been isolated from the facial nerve in some patients with Bell's palsy. Due to these possible etiologies, all of the medicines above may be of some use. Current summaries of randomized, controlled trials indicate that prednisone and/or acyclovir may provide a slightly higher chance of complete recovery, although other trials indicate no difference in long-term outcomes of patients given placebo versus treatment. Lubrication is beneficial to protect the cornea if a patient is unable to completely close the affected eye, especially at night.

95–A

The most serious initial consequence of Bell's palsy is corneal abrasion, which may result from inability to completely close the eye due to weakness of the orbicularis muscle. Lubricating the eye, as well as taping shut the lid at night may be needed to protect the eye. If the eye shows evidence of corneal abrasion by fluorescein stain, or if lid weakness persists for two to three weeks, consider referral to ophthalmology.

96–B

Bell's palsy affects men and women almost equally; peak incidence is between ages 10 and 40. It is equal between right and left sides of the face. Incidence is 23/100,000 people per year or 1/60 to 70 people per lifetime.

97–A

Antihypertensive medications should be chosen based on each particular patient. In the patient with diabetes and chronic renal insufficiency with proteinuria, an ACE inhibitor should be first-line therapy. ACE inhibitors have been proven to slow the progression of renal disease in these patients. An ARB could be used if the patient were not able to tolerate ACE inhibitors due to cough or angioedema. A potassium-sparing diuretic would be a good choice in a patient with CHF, but would not be appropriate in the patient with renal insufficiency due to risk of hyperkalemia. A calcium channel blocker would be a good agent in a patient with diastolic dysfunction, atrial fibrillation with rapid ventricular response, or angina.

ANSWERS

98–D

Noncompliance with antihypertensive medications (especially clonidine with effects of rebound hypertension) could have caused this emergency. Cocaine use undoubtedly could cause hypertensive effects. Over-the-counter decongestants and cough syrups may contain pseudoephedrine, which can elevate blood pressure. Cannabis does not contribute to hypertension.

99–A

The image in (a) shows blurred disc margins and hyperemic vessels, consistent with a diagnosis of a swollen optic nerve; papilledema is defined as swollen optic nerves in the presence of increased intracranial pressure. The image in (b) reveals a sharp disc with superior-temporal flame-shaped hemorrhages and cotton wool spots in the distribution of the superior vein; note the dilated vein. The image in (b) is consistent with a diagnosis of a branch retinal vein occlusion, which can be caused by HTN, microvascular disease, and hypercoagulable states. The image in (c) shows a massive preretinal hemorrhage with overlying fibrosis, consistent with a vitreous hemorrhage; may be caused by trauma, or neovascularization (DM, sickle cell, sarcoid). The image in (d) shows a blurred central macula with gray flecks, consistent with central serous retinopathy. This occurs in young males with Type A personalities or recent emotional stress; can also occur with high systemic prednisone use.

100–C

Treatment of a hypertensive emergency requires parenteral therapy for rapid onset, and ease of titration to goal BP. BP should be lowered at most by 25% in the first two hours, then toward 160/100 within six hours. By definition, treatment is based upon end-organ damage, not by the BP value. Intravenous nitroprusside is the preferred agent, but other IV agents can be used (nitroglycerin, labetalol, enalapril).

101–B

Neurocardiogenic syncope was previously called vasovagal syncope. It is characterized by initial sympathetic overstimulation (which may cause dilated pupils, sweating, yawning, and possible tachycardia) followed by interruption of the sympathetic response, which causes bradycardia, hypotension, and hypoperfusion. The myocardium is normal and the prognosis is excellent. Upright tilt-testing may produce both the premonitory symptoms and the resultant syncope or near-syncope. It is treated with beta-blockers to block the initial sympathetic over-stimulation.

102–C

Patients with cardiac-origin syncope (valvular disease, ischemic heart disease, and dysrhythmias) have an average one-year mortality of 25%, whereas non-cardiac origin (all others including neurocardiogenic syncope) confers an 8–9% annual mortality risk.

103–D

Holter monitoring can be helpful in the patient with sudden onset of syncope without warning. It does not always correlate to symptoms; patients may have PVCs, beats of v-tach, or sinus pauses and feel no symptoms. In some patients, an "event monitor" is more telling. It records the previous two to five minutes of cardiac activity once a symptom is felt and recorded by the patient. An echocardiogram would be helpful in the patient with a heart murmur or click or effort-induced syncope. An exercise stress test cannot only unmask coronary artery disease but may provoke an arrhythmia that has been undetected thus far. A V/Q scan is used to measure ventilation and perfusion of the lungs and would not be helpful in this setting.

104–D

Meniere's disease is associated with hearing loss, tinnitus, and ear pressure with vertigo; it can usually be diagnosed by history, and treatment includes bed rest and anticholinergics (like meclizine). Acute labyrinthitis is a postviral effect on the cochlea and labyrinth and is also accompanied by tinnitus and hearing loss. Acoustic neuroma may present with vague vertiginous symptoms with hearing loss and tinnitus but is progressive and causes a decreased corneal reflex fairly early on; MRI is needed to diagnose this problem. Benign positional vertigo can be diagnosed by history and provocative physical exam; it is common in the elderly and usually resolves completely within six months.

105–C

Although sedentary lifestyle does confer an increased risk of coronary artery disease, obesity (BMI >27) is not classified as a major risk factor. Nonmodifiable risk factors are age, sex, and

ANSWERS

family history. Modifiable risk factors are diabetes, smoking, hypertension, and hyperlipidemia.

106–A

For coronary artery disease, the primary goal is to achieve an LDL of <100. Ideally, HDL will also rise to above 50 and the total cholesterol will fall.

107–D

Although the NCEP guidelines do recommend routine screening for all adults even without risk factors, the significance of a nonfasting cholesterol

110–A

All but 5% of COPD cases are due to smoking; second-hand smoke and air pollution may factor into many of those minority cases. Smoking cessation will revert decline in lung function to values of non-smokers.

111–C

Scheduled use of beta-agonists regardless of symptoms is not beneficial for mild, intermittent asthma (should be used on as-needed basis only). Note: all MDIs should be used with a spacer!

TABLE A111. Types of Asthma				
TYPE OF ASTHMA	DEFINITION	BASAL CONTROL	AS-NEEDED MEDICINES	CONSIDER
Mild intermittent	Symptoms less than weekly with normal lung function	None	Short-acting beta-agonists + anti-cholinergic	
Mild persistent	Symptoms more than weekly, less than daily with normal lung function	Low-dose inhaled steroid (or cromolyn/nedocromil in kids)	Short-acting beta-agonists + anti-cholinergic	Leukotriene modifier
Exercise induced	Exacerbation triggered reproducibly by exercise	Same as mild persistent	Short-acting beta-agonist prior to exercise	
Moderate persistent	Daily symptoms with mild to moderate variable airflow obstruction	Inhaled steroid plus second agent	Short-acting beta-agonist, anti-cholinergic, oral steroid	Long-acting beta-agonist, leukotriene inhibitor
Severe	Daily symptoms, frequent night symptoms, moderate to severe variable airflow obstruction	Inhaled steroid, long-acting beta-agonist, leukotriene modifier	Short-acting beta-agonist, anti-cholinergic, oral steroids	Oral steroids

plus HDL only in this low-risk patient is debatable. Certainly the daughter would benefit from diet/exercise education and follow-up fasting cholesterol levels at some point in the future.

108–B

Any patient who has had a reaction of angioedema to any drug should not be tried on an ACE inhibitor, due to the increased possibility of angioedema to the ACE.

109–D

For a pure COPD exacerbation, inhaled corticosteroids have not been shown to be beneficial. Inhaled beta agonists, inhaled anticholinergics, treatment of underlying bronchitis with antibiotics, and oral corticosteroids have been shown to modify the course of the exacerbation. Long-term management of COPD also includes oxygen in patients with chronic hypoxemia, mucolytics, and cessation of smoking.

112–A

Decreased FEV-1 (amount of air blown out in one second) will be seen with the obstruction of COPD and asthma. In asthma without significant inflammation or mucus plugging, the FEV-1 should increase 12% and more than 200 mL post-bronchodilator to be significant. DLCO (diffusing capacity) will be decreased in emphysema, which causes the destruction of alveolar units and pulmonary capillaries. Intracardiac shunts will increase the DLCO due to increased pulmonary blood flow. Usually, an increased DLCO on PFTs is not clinically significant.

113–B

This patient is a tuberculin converter, a contact of a household converter. The new term for this is "latent TB infection"; she is at high risk as a recent converter and needs treatment with INH for six to nine months. Nine months of INH is the new standard recommendation for all patients with LTBI, and it is the only acceptable regimen for patients under age 18. Nine months of treatment confers a higher rate of clearing the infection; six months is an acceptable but inferior option for otherwise low-risk patients. (Clearance rates are 69% for six months and 93% for 12 months.) If her father had active tuberculosis, she would need INH even with a negative PPD. She should be questioned for risk factors for HIV. She doesn't need a PPD at any time in the future (it will be positive). All household contacts need to be screened and treated if PPD-positive.

114–D

In April 2000, the CDC changed their guidelines regarding monitoring for toxicity with INH therapy. Most people can tolerate INH without difficulty. The INH-associated hepatitis is related to age; however, because of its low incidence, routine LFTs are not indicated just due to age of the patient.

TABLE A114. Percent of INH-Taking Patients Who Develop Hepatitis by Age	
AGE	HEPATITIS
<20 years	0.0%
20–34	0.3%
35–49	1.2%
50–64	2.3%
>64	0.8%

All patients taking INH should be seen monthly face-to-face and questioned about toxicity, as well as suggestive symptoms (nausea, jaundice, numbness, rashes, fatigue). Only one month of INH should be given at a time to ensure follow-up. Baseline and monthly LFTs are recommended only in HIV infection, drug injection, pregnancy, postpartum women of color (African-Americans and Hispanic women have a greater risk of hepatitis), and alcoholism or liver disease.

115–A

Pyridoxine (B6) can help prevent the neuropathic side effects of INH. It should be given to patients at high risk for peripheral neuropathy (diabetes, uremia, alcoholism, malnutrition, HIV infection, advanced age), and also pregnancy and seizure disorder. Otherwise healthy children are not at high risk for neuropathy.

116–B

In most cases BCG history can be ignored. PPD reactions over 10 mm are unusual several years after vaccination. In cases of recent (<1 year)

vaccination, the PPD can be repeated in one year before deciding on treatment.

117–B

Digoxin levels do not need to be monitored in patients who are taking the medication for atrial fibrillation; therapeutic levels are measured according to its effects, specifically, rate control. In patients who take digoxin for congestive heart failure, however, serum levels must be monitored to maintain therapeutic levels.

118–D

Early electrical cardioversion is indicated in patients with atrial fibrillation who are hemodynamically unstable or experiencing myocardial ischemia, and in stable patients with duration of atrial fibrillation less than 48 hours. The last patient is not a candidate for *early* electrical cardioversion, but may receive cardioversion after completing a three to four week course of anticoagulation, and a transesophageal echocardiogram excluding an atrial thrombus.

119–C

In patients with valvular dysfunction due to rheumatic heart disease, the incidence is 85% mitral valve, 22% aortic valve, 10–16% tricuspid valve, and rare pulmonic valve.

120–D

The atrial rate in atrial fibrillation ranges between 400 and 600 beats/minute.

121–C

The most important active compound in cigarette smoke contributing to addiction is nicotine. Nicotine withdrawal is associated with a syndrome of irritability, bradycardia, trouble sleeping, anxiety, impaired concentration, impaired reaction time, restlessness, hunger, weight gain, impotence, and depression.

122–C

Smoking cessation intervention includes

1) pharmacologic therapy:
   a) nicotine replacement: patch, gum, spray, inhaler
   b) bupropion
2) behavioral therapy:
   a) support groups
   b) hypnotherapy
   c) cognitive behavior therapy

ANSWERS

Studies have shown that all of the above improve quit rates when compared with placebo.

Pharmacologic therapies approximately double quit rates when compared with placebo. Contraindications to nicotine replacement therapy include pregnancy, recent MI, arrhythmia, unstable angina, and vasospastic disease. Nicotine spray is good for highly dependent smokers, and the inhaler mimics the hand-to-mouth behavior of smoking. Combining nicotine replacement with bupropion has been shown to improve quit rates in recent studies:

TABLE A122. Smoking Cessation Rates When Adding Bupropion

NICOTINE REPLACEMENT	QUIT RATE	ADDING BUPROPION
Gum	23% at 12 weeks	34% at 12 weeks
	15% at 24 weeks	28% at 24 weeks
Spray	35% at 6 weeks	51% at 6 weeks
	25% at 12 weeks	37% at 12 weeks

Contraindications to bupropion include a history of seizures, concurrent MAOI use, eating disorders, heavy alcohol use, or a history of head trauma in the past.

The most aggressive behavioral programs achieve quit rates of 20%, and these quit rates can also be augmented by the addition of pharmacologic therapy.

123–A

The lifetime incidence for major depression is remarkably high, averaging 7–12% for men and 20–25% for women. Commonly accepted criteria for major depression include the presence of five or more of the following for the previous two weeks: depressed mood, loss of interest or pleasure, weight loss or gain, insomnia or hypersomnia, psychomotor agitation or retardation, fatigue and loss of energy, feelings of worthlessness or guilt, decreased ability to concentrate or think, and recurrent thoughts of death or suicidal ideation.

124–B

SSRIs are generally considered the treatment of choice for depression. Their efficacy is comparable to that of TCAs, but they do not exert the same cholinergic and sedative effects, are not as lethal in overdose, are easier to administer, and are well-tolerated. Psychotherapy has been found to be close in efficacy to antidepressants; however, it has slower onset of action and recurrence of depression is common.

TABLE A124-1. Patient-Based Characteristics in Choosing an SSRI

ANXIETY	INSOMNIA	ANXIETY, OCD, PTSD	TOBACCO, DRUG CESSATION
nefazodone	nefazodone	paroxetine	bupropion
paroxetine	mirtazapine	sertraline	
mirtazapine	paroxetine	fluvoxamine	
citalopram	fluvoxamine	citalopram	
venlafaxine	citalopram	fluoxetine	
		nefazodone	

(Note: there is a new black box warning of liver failure and related deaths in patients on nefazodone.)

TABLE A124-2. Choosing an Antidepressant

DRUG CLASS	PROS	CONS
TCA	• very effective • also for pain, fibromyalgia, migraine	• high incidence of side effects (SE) • less cost-effective 2° labs, dose titration • avoid in BPH, urinary retention, dementia, cardiac conduction disease, closed angle glaucoma
MAOI	• useful for Rx-resistant patients • no anticholinergic SE	• orthostatic hypotension • dietary restrictions • drug interactions • lethal in OD
Bupropion	• no anticholinergic SE • few GI SE, no weight gain • minimal sexual SE • useful for ADHD, cocaine abuse, smoking cessation • no withdrawal symptoms	• 0.1–0.4% incidence seizures w/immediate-acting form only • not for panic d/o, PTSD, OCD
SSRI	• very effective • easy to prescribe • favorable SE profile • safe in OD • many psych applications	• weight gain w/chronic use • sexual and GI SE • transient withdrawal symptoms
Mirtazapine	• no sexual SE • no insomnia, anxiety • may help severe depression	• significant sedation, dry mouth • significant weight gain • possible increase in TG, cholesterol levels • 1.1/1000 incidence agranulocytosis

125–C

Length of anticoagulation for first-time DVT has been studied extensively and is still somewhat controversial. What is clear is that at least three months of anticoagulation is necessary to reduce recurrence risk and to lower morbidity and mortality. It is not necessary to anticoagulate for life for an otherwise uncomplicated first-time DVT.

126–B

Increasing the INR beyond 3 greatly increases complications of anticoagulation without decreasing morbidity and mortality of DVT. Most anticoagulation therapy is aimed at the goal INR of 2–3, with the exception of auto-immune disorders like anti-cardiolipin antibody and the hypercoagulable syndrome of lupus, which require anti-coagulation to an INR between 3 and 4.

127–A

A nondiagnostic ultrasound in the face of an abnormal physical exam shouldn't totally reassure you. This type of patient is more likely to have a distal or isolated calf vein thrombosis, which although it is not able to cause pulmonary embolism immediately, has a 50% chance of extending proximally. Venography, although the gold standard, is invasive, painful, difficult to obtain, and 25% of the time is unsuccessful. D-dimers can be helpful in ruling out the presence of a clot if they are normal, but the accurate version of the test may not be offered at your institution. This patient deserves extensive counseling on worsening signs and symptoms, and a timely follow-up ultrasound.

128–D

The options of inpatient versus outpatient treatment should be carefully considered for each patient. Inpatient treatment may be necessary for the patient with significant co-morbidities or who is marginally housed. It will take your patient six to eight days to become therapeutic on Coumadin (at which point the heparin of choice can be discontinued). Hospitalized patients receiving IV unfractionated heparin should have their blood count followed to assess for heparin-induced thrombocytopenia. Protamine sulfate may be used to reverse unfractionated heparin in an emergency. LMWH can be used in isolation for the duration of treatment if preferred by the patient/provider. The advantage of LMWH is that it doesn't need to be monitored (and is difficult to monitor); however, that can cause complications. The usual dose of 1mg/kg subcutaneous twice a day (treatment dose) has not been tested over weights of 100 kg; the effect may be variable. As with any anticoagulation, recent or current major hemorrhage (intracranial, retroperitoneal, joint, or muscle bleeding) is a contraindication to use. Heparin is excreted renally; in renal failure the effect may

be variable and the PT/PTT must be monitored. Diabetics could be excellent candidates for outpatient treatment, as they are already familiar with needle technique. Patients taking Coumadin need extensive education as to dietary and medicinal interactions; the PT should be measured every one to two weeks until stable and then monthly.

129–D

Since pernicious anemia is caused by vitamin B12 malabsorption, it must be administered intramuscularly. There is no replacement intrinsic factor available. Oral folic acid will not correct the vitamin B12 deficiency.

130–D

Zidovudine administration will cause a macrocytic anemia, but is not a cause of vitamin B12 deficiency or megaloblastic anemia. Infestation with *Diphyllobothrium latum* competes for vitamin B12 in the gut and can cause deficiency. Animal products are the only dietary source of cobalamin: meat and dairy. Gastrectomy will impair absorption of vitamin B12 because intrinsic factor is secreted by gastric parietal cells.

131–A

Hypersegmented neutrophils is a characteristic finding that should raise the suspicion for a megaloblastic anemia like pernicious anemia. Ringed sideroblasts (rings within the RBCs) is a finding in sideroblastic anemia (ineffective erythropoiesis usually due to toxins like alcohol or lead). Sickle-shaped RBCs are found in sickle cell anemia. Band neutrophils (immature neutrophils) with Dohle bodies (aggregates of rough endoplasmic reticulum) are found in infections and other toxic states.

132–B

Neurologic abnormalities are not found in megaloblastic anemia secondary to folic acid deficiency; they only occur in vitamin B12 deficiency. It is imperative that the physician NOT treat empirically with folic acid for a megaloblastic anemia, as an untreated vitamin B12 deficiency will lead to worsening, irreversible neurologic abnormalities. Poor nutritional state, pallor, tachycardia, cheilosis, and glossitis are all signs and symptoms in a folic acid deficiency.

ANSWERS

133–B

The increasing incidence and prevalence of CHF is attributed to the decreasing mortality from acute myocardial infarctions. Ischemic heart disease is the primary etiology, followed by hypertension and other dilated cardiomyopathies (alcohol, viral, idiopathic). CHF morbidity and mortality in African-Americans is more than twice that for Caucasians, likely due to differences in the prevalence of hypertension and diabetes, and differences in access to care.

134–C

A split S1 is physiologic, composed by the mitral valve closure, and then the later tricuspid valve closure; heard loudest at the lower left sternal border, but difficult to auscultate secondary to the loud mitral sound; does not vary with respiration. A split S2 is also physiologic, composed of the aortic valve sound, and then the pulmonic valve sound; varies with inspiration. An S3 gallop is characteristic of CHF as blood flows from the left atrium into the left ventricle in early diastole. An S4 is the sound of atrial contraction (atrial kick), often heard after a myocardial infarction.

135–D

Angiotensin receptor blockers (ARBs) have not yet been studied in large clinical trials for use in CHF. Trials in smaller studies show a poorer survival rate with losartan; therefore, ARBs are not routinely used to treat systolic dysfunction CHF. Loop diuretics (furosemide) effectively attenuate CHF symptoms (pulmonary and peripheral edema). Angiotensin converting enzyme inhibitors (ACE-inhibitors) reduce afterload, thereby improving pump function and cardiac output. Beta-blockers and potassium-sparing diuretics block the neurohumoral activation of catecholamine release and sodium retention, thereby improving cardiac function.

136–D

Afterload reduction (using ACE-inhibitors and hydralazine with nitrates) and neurohumoral blockade (using beta-blockers and potassium-sparing diuretics) have all shown mortality benefit in CHF. Loop diuretics prove to be effective in symptom control, but there have been no studies examining survival.

ACE-inhibitors: CONSENSUS trial, SOLVD trial
Beta-blockers: CIBIS-II trial, MERIT trial
Potassium-sparing diuretics: RALES trial

137–D

Colchicine is the only listed medication that should be used for an acute attack of gout. It works by inhibiting neutrophil migration, and can be administered IV or by mouth during an acute attack. Side effects of oral administration are nausea, vomiting, and diarrhea. Colchicine at lower doses is also indicated for prevention of attacks during the intercritical phase of gout. Allopurinol, an analog of hypoxanthine, competitively inhibits xanthine oxidase, thereby decreasing the synthesis of uric acid. Probenecid and sulfinpyrazone increase urinary excretion of uric acid by blocking its tubular reabsorption. Allopurinol and uricosuric agents should be avoided during acute attacks because fluctuations in the serum uric acid concentration can prolong the episode. They are important treatment options, however, in chronic gout. Aspirin is not a treatment option for gout attacks, and may in fact increase serum uric acid concentrations by decreasing tubular excretion of urate. Other treatment choices during acute gouty episodes are NSAIDs (with the exception of ASA) and corticosteroids.

138–A

Arthrocentesis during an attack would not be useful in determining treatment for a patient with tophaceous gout. A patient with tophaceous gout has chronic gout, with many years of episodic or constant hyperuricemia leading to deposition of urate crystals on osseous, articular, cartilaginous and soft tissue areas—pinna of the ears, ulnar surface of the forearms, Achilles tendons. Tests that would be useful are a serum uric acid level and a 24-hour urine collection test for uric acid to determine whether the patient is an overproducer of uric acid or an underexcreter of uric acid. The results would allow the physician to decide whether to treat with allopurinol to inhibit synthesis, or with a uricosuric agent to increase excretion. The creatinine clearance is also necessary as patients with impaired creatinine clearance or renal function would not be prescribed uricosuric agents. (Of note, determining the serum uric acid level would not be useful in an acute attack, as it may be normal, and an elevated serum uric acid level alone is not specific for gout.)

139–E

Taking ibuprofen would help to treat a gout attack, not trigger one. Trauma, alcohol use, infection, emotional stress, and dietary indiscretions may precipitate attacks. Diuretics and aspirin decrease urinary excretion of urate by interfering with its tubular transport, and thereby increase serum uric acid levels.

140–C

Tophi and chronic inflammation of joints are clinical features of chronic gout. Bony erosion can be demonstrated in radiographs of involved joints. Nephrolithiasis is a common presentation of renal involvement; however, stones will be composed of uric acid, which are radiolucent. Radiopaque stones are composed of calcium phosphate, calcium oxalate, cysteine, and struvite, and are not caused by gout.

141–D

Osteoarthritis is defined as the loss of articular cartilage with associated remodeling of subchondral bone, resulting in sclerosis, subchondral bone collapse, bone cysts, and osteophyte formation. The pathogenesis is not precisely known; however, it is related to abnormal mechanics (failure of cartilage related to excessive load-bearing across a joint) or biologic failure (inability of cells to respond to joint stress).

In contrast to rheumatoid arthritis or other connective tissue diseases, inflammation is not a prominent finding in osteoarthritis, and therefore signs of prominent inflammation such as joint effusions and localized warmth should suggest another etiology.

142–A

Osteoarthritis most commonly affects the hands, spine, knees, and hips. In many cases only a single joint is involved; however, it is also common to have generalized osteoarthritis, which is characterized by the involvement of three or more areas, especially the distal and proximal interphalangeal joints of the hands, the first metatarsophalangeal and first carpometacarpal joints, the knees, the cervical and lumbar spine, and the hips.

143–D

Currently, there is no gold standard diagnostic test, and diagnosis is based on history, PE findings, and x-ray findings.

Symptoms and exam findings suggestive of osteoarthritis include deep, aching pain which is poorly localized and occurs with use, joint stiffness in the mornings which rarely exceeds 30 minutes duration, crepitus on motion, limitation of joint motion, and giving way of weight-bearing joints.

X-ray findings of osteoarthritis include joint space narrowing and osteophyte formation, and correlate poorly with clinical symptoms; only 30% of patients with x-ray evidence of osteoarthritis complain of pain.

The American College of Rheumatology criteria for diagnosis of osteoarthritis of the knee require:

1) knee pain
2) radiographic osteophytes
3) at least one of the following: age over 50 years, morning stiffness for less than 30 minutes, crepitus

144–B

Management of osteoarthritis requires a multifaceted approach. The keystone of overall therapy is nonpharmacologic, most important of which are exercise programs and weight-loss strategies for the obese. Other nonpharmacologic approaches include self-management programs, physical therapy with range of motion and strengthening exercises, assisted devices for ambulation, thermal therapy, and joint protection.

Pharmacologic management of osteoarthritis can help reduce pain and prevent disability.

- initial drug of choice: acetaminophen—*if inadequate proceed to→*
  - NSAIDs (especially if there is some inflammation on top of the OA)
  - topical capsaicin
  - chondroitin, glucosamine
  - intra-articular hyaluronic acid
  - intra-articular steroids
  - arthroscopy
  - joint replacement

145–B

Calcium-containing stones constitute approximately 75% of kidney stones; of which 30–35% are calcium oxalate, 5% are calcium phosphate, and 30–35% are mixed calcium oxalate and calcium phosphate. 5–10% are uric acid stones, 2% are cysteine stones, and 15–20% are struvite stones (magnesium ammonium phosphate, or "triple stones").

ANSWERS

146–C

Magnesium ammonium phosphate ("triple stones" or struvite) stones are a result of recurrent UTI by urease-producing bacteria, such as *Proteus*, *Providencia*, *Klebsiella*, *Pseudomonas*, *Serratia*, and *Enterobacter*. This patient has had several UTIs, the current episode with *Proteus*. Her urine pH is 8, which is consistent with the alkaline urine of struvite stones. Urea is degraded into NH_3 and CO_2 by urease. When the NH_3 hydrolyzes to NH_4^+, the pH rises to 8 or 9, and the presence of NH_4^+ precipitates out both magnesium and phosphate, thus forming the triple stones. Most kidney stones occur in men; the exception is struvite, which is most commonly found in women. These stones are also known as staghorn calculi given their characteristic appearance shaped by the molding of the renal pelvis and calyxes.

147–D

Focal glomerulosclerosis is an idiopathic nephrotic syndrome unrelated to pyelonephritis. Renal scarring secondary to chronic pyelonephritis can lead to renin-mediated hypertension, as well as renal insufficiency. Renal or perinephric abscesses can develop secondary to unrelieved obstruction. Xanthogranulomatous pyelonephritis is the development of a granuloma secondary to chronic bacterial infection, usually *Proteus mirabilis*; nephrolithiasis has occurred in the majority of patients with this complication.

148–C

Renal tuberculosis classically presents as sterile pyuria.

149–B

Finasteride, a 5-α reductase inhibitor, acts by blocking the conversion of testosterone to dihydrotestosterone. Flutamide is a nonsteroidal antiandrogen whose proposed mechanism of action is the competitive binding of the dihydrotestosterone receptor. Leuprolide is a luteinizing hormone-releasing hormone agonist (LHRH agonist). Doxazosin is a treatment for BPH, not prostate cancer. It is an α_1 blocker that relaxes smooth muscle in the prostate neck and bladder base to relieve obstructive urinary symptoms.

All treatments for prostate cancer are aimed at blocking testosterone, from the hypothalamic-pituitary axis, to the adrenal glands, to the testes.

TABLE A149. Treatments for Prostate Cancer		
LEVEL	TREATMENT MODALITY	MECHANISM OF ACTION
Hypothalamic-pituitary	Leuprolide	LHRH agonist
Adrenal	Glucocorticoids Ketoconazole	Ablation of adrenal production of androgens
Testes	Finasteride	5-α reductase inhibitor that blocks the conversion of testosterone to dihydrotestosterone
	Orchiectomy	Removal of circulating testosterone by ablation of testes
Prostate	Flutamide	Nonsteroidal antiandrogen that blocks the uptake and nuclear binding of androgens in target tissues

150–A

Biopsy of a nodule is not a screening test; it would be a diagnostic test of an abnormality. Screening tests for prostate cancer are the digital rectal examination, serum prostate-specific antigen (PSA) level, and transrectal ultrasound of the prostate.

151–D

Past history of osteopenia is not a risk factor for falls in the elderly, but is a risk factor for the development of vertebral fractures. Elimination of throw rugs in the home can reduce the risk of falls in the elderly. Many drugs can increase the risk for falls in the elderly, such as diuretics, antihistamines, antihypertensives—ophthalmologic agents are often overlooked, but timolol is a β-blocker that can yield systemic effects which increase fall risk. Presbyopia and any decreased visual acuity will increase fall risk.

152–C

The majority of prostate carcinomas are adenocarcinomas. Most arise in the peripheral zone of the prostate. The likelihood of metastases is increased in patients with less well-differentiated and larger adenocarcinomas. Transitional cell carcinoma is the most common histopathology of bladder carcinomas. Clear cell carcinomas are adenocarcinomas most commonly found in adult renal tumors (also known as hypernephromas, renal cell carcinoma, or Grawitz's tumor). Seminomas are testicular tumors.

153–D

The offending agent is ibuprofen. It should be discontinued at this time. Furosemide can be held, but should ultimately be continued in this patient with symptomatic CHF. Emergent hemodialysis is not warranted in the asymptomatic patient with acute renal failure. The patient should continue to receive antibiotics to treat pneumonia, but the dose must be adjusted for his renal failure and creatinine clearance.

154–B

Treatment modalities for hyperkalemia are calcium gluconate to stabilize the myocardium, especially in a patient with EKG changes, sodium bicarbonate (intracellular shift of potassium), administration of insulin and glucose (intracellular shift), inhaled beta-agonist therapy (intracellular shift), Kayexalate (GI excretion of potassium via gutbinders), and hemodialysis. Magnesium gluconate would be a treatment option for hypokalemia. (Mnemonic: C BIG K Drop: calcium gluconate, bicarbonate, beta-agonists, insulin and glucose, Kayexalate, dialysis.)

155–C

Many medications need dose adjustment in renal insufficiency, including antibiotics, antivirals, antituberculosis medications, hypoglycemic agents, and other renally excreted medications. Acetaminophen, thiamine, multivitamins, and folic acid do not require adjustment.

156–C

Indications for emergent hemodialysis are remembered by the mnemonic: AEIOU (severe acidosis, electrolyte imbalances, ingestions, fluid overload, and uremia). The patient in (a) is certainly acidemic, but this acidosis is of respiratory origin; given his obtunded state, high pCO_2, and normal pO_2 on oxygen therapy, this patient is retaining CO_2, with a depressed respiratory drive (no longer hypoxic). The treatment is discontinuation of O_2 therapy and intubation if gas exchange does not improve. The patient in (b) has chronic renal insufficiency/failure; he will probably require long-term hemodialysis in the future, but the BUN and creatinine levels alone

do not mandate emergent hemodialysis. The patient in (c) will likely require emergent hemodialysis given the ingestion of salicylates, which cause a metabolic acidosis. The patient in (d) is hyperkalemic but asymptomatic without EKG changes and a clear underlying cause of the electrolyte disturbance. Spironolactone should be discontinued, and other temporizing measures as noted above may be attempted first.

157–A

Abscess formation is a feature of Crohn's disease, not ulcerative colitis.

TABLE A157. Comparison of Crohn's Disease and Ulcerative Colitis

	CROHN'S DISEASE	ULCERATIVE COLITIS
Diarrhea	Non-bloody	Bloody
Pathology	Transmural inflammation	• Mucosal and submucosal inflammation • Microabscesses in the crypts of Lieberkuhn
Pattern of lesions	Skip lesions	Continuous lesions
Location	Any segment of the GI tract from mouth to anus	Limited to colon
Complications	• Fistulas • Abscesses • Strictures	• Severe anemia due to hemorrhage • Toxic megacolon
Extraintestinal manifestations	• Dermatologic: erythema nodosum, pyoderma gangrenosum, episcleritis, keratoconjunctivitis • Sclerosing cholangitis • Arthritis • **Renal disease only found in Crohn's disease** • Urolithiasis: calcium oxalate stones secondary to increased oxalate absorption; uric acid stones secondary to increased cell turnover and acidic urine	• Dermatologic: erythema nodosum, pyoderma gangrenosum, episcleritis, keratoconjunctivitis • Sclerosing cholangitis • Arthritis
Cancer risk	+	+++

158–C

Urolithiasis. See Table A157.

ANSWERS

159–A

Erythema nodosum. Both erythema nodosum and pyoderma gangrenosum are extraintestinal manifestations of IBD; erythema nodosum is more commonly found.

160–D

Skip lesions. See Table A157.

161–B

7. The Glasgow coma scale is based upon three categories: eye opening, verbal response, and motor response. The minimum score is 3, and the maximum score is 14, when the score for each category is added together.

TABLE A161. The Glasgow Coma Scale		
Eye opening	Spontaneous	4
	To speech	3
	To pain	2
	None	1
Verbal response	Oriented	5
	Confused	4
	Inappropriate words	3
	Incomprehensible sounds	2
	None	1
Motor response	Localizes pain/obeys commands	5
	Withdraws to pain	4
	Flexor response to pain (cerebrate posturing)	3
	Extensor response to pain (decorticate posturing)	2
	None	1

This patient has a score of 7:1 (no eye opening) + 2 (incomprehensible sounds) + 4 (withdrawal from painful stimuli).

162–C

The most likely cause is hepatic encephalopathy secondary to this patient's acute upper GI bleed causing increased protein load in his gut, with subsequent development of coma. Serum ammonia levels may be elevated, but have a poor correlation with symptomatology. Spontaneous bacterial peritonitis (SBP) is common in patients with ascites in end stage liver disease, but this patient does not exhibit these signs or symptoms (fever, peritoneal signs on abdominal exam, ascites); also a patient with SBP would not be in a coma. Hepatorenal syndrome is also a complication in patients with end stage liver disease, but this would present with acute renal failure—oliguria and anuria; coma is possible in later stages of hepatorenal syndrome secondary to uremia, but not acutely as in this patient. An ischemic cerebrovascular accident is not likely in this patient.

163–D

Hepatomegaly is uncommon in end stage liver cirrhosis, as the liver is commonly fibrotic and shrunken. Common physical examination findings are malnutrition, coagulopathy with easy bruising, petechiae, spider telangiectasias, caput medusa, fetor hepaticus, jaundice, pruritus, ascites, and asterixis.

164–A

Placement of a femoral catheter is not appropriate for intravenous fluid resuscitation (caveat: unless other access cannot be obtained). Two large-bore (14 Ga. or 16 Ga.) peripheral catheters should be placed as shorter peripheral lines afford more rapid infusion than longer central lines. Ideal solutions for rapid intravenous fluid resuscitation are normal saline or lactated Ringer's solution.

165–B

Alcohol withdrawal seizures (generalized and nonfocal seizures) occur less than 48 hours from the last drink. If a seizure occurs outside that time frame, is a first-time seizure, or is associated with trauma or fever, it should be worked up.

166–C

Lorazepam (Ativan) may be given by mouth, intravenously, or intramuscularly. Chlordiazepoxide (Librium) and diazepam (Valium) are absorbed erratically intramuscularly and can be associated with sterile abscess.

167–A

25 mg chlordiazepoxide is equivalent to 1–2 mg lorazepam by mouth. Lorazepam is preferable in the elderly and those with liver disease, as chlordiazepoxide and diazepam can accumulate. It is always preferable to use one drug in one route when treating alcohol withdrawal, as the different onsets of action and half-lives of the drugs affect the clinical picture.

168–B

Mortality of DTs approaches 5%, commonly from pneumonia, arrhythmia, or other complications.

169–D

A DNR/DNI order does not exclude treatment for reversible causes; this patient's illness is easily reversible with the appropriate treatment. Patients with advanced directives should still be treated as any other patient, except for the specific orders noted. In discussing an advanced directive with a patient or the patient's DPOA (durable power of attorney) for healthcare, it is more important to understand and clarify the patient's values and beliefs regarding independence, being free of pain, cognitive state, affect of their illness or state on the family (ideas about burdening the family, or causing suffering for the family), rather than trying to delineate all possibilities of treatment options available at the end of life.

170–B

ADLs (activities of daily living) include bathing, dressing, eating, transferring from bed to chair, toileting, and continence. IADLs (instrumental activities of daily living) include transportation, shopping, cooking, using the telephone, managing money, taking medications, housecleaning, and doing laundry.

171–A

Urge incontinence, caused by detrusor instability, is the most common type of incontinence in the elderly. Stress incontinence is second most common in elderly women, while overflow incontinence is second most common in elderly men. Incontinence is prevalent in the elderly: 25% in community dwelling elderly, 50% in those hospitalized, 75% in nursing home residents. Women are affected twice as often as men. It is an underreported problem, and should be asked of all elderly patients.

172–C

Primary prevention targets the prevention of disease from occurring. Secondary prevention tries to detect disease while a patient is still asymptomatic, in the hopes that early intervention may alter the course of the disease. Tertiary prevention attempts to limit the impact of a known disease. Home safety guidance, smoking cessation and exercise counseling, and immunizations (pneumococcal vaccination) are all primary prevention measures. Colorectal cancer screening is a type of secondary prevention.

173–C

The body mass index is a standardized measure that is highly correlated with body fat. It is defined as weight in kilograms divided by height in meters squared (kg/m^2). People with BMIs between 25 and 30 are characterized as overweight, those with BMIs above 30 are characterized as obese, and those with BMI greater than 40 are characterized as morbidly obese.

174–D

According to the NIH, 55% of U.S. women have a BMI of 25 and above ("overweight"), while 20% of men and 25% of women are "obese" (BMI >30).

175–C

One pound of fat loss results from a 3500 calorie deficit. Thus a diet restriction of 500 calories per day will result in one pound of weight loss per week, given the same caloric expenditure.

176–A

Pharmacologic treatment of obesity has a troubled history in the United States. Functional morbidity and mortality have not been examined as outcome measures; sustained weight loss is the usual assessment tool. Fenfluramine and dexfenfluramine have been associated with valvular heart disease and pulmonary hypertension. Phenylpropanolamine has been associated with increased risk of hemorrhagic stroke. Sibutramine and phentermine (centrally acting agents) may help promote modest weight loss in obese people, but weight regain is likely after treatment is stopped and long-term safety data is not available. Orlistat (interferes with GI fat absorption) may assist efforts at modest weight loss, but it also has significant unpleasant side effects and hasn't undergone long-term studies. Many other pharmacologic interventions are being studied.

177–C

The true sensitivity of the Hemoccult II test for colon cancer and large bleeding polyps is likely 50%; estimates range from 37% to 69%. It is less sensitive for smaller polyps and must be repeated every one to two years. Approximately 75–90% of positive test results are false-positives (the positive predictive value is approximately 20%).

178–B

Specificity is the proportion of people without the disease who have a negative test. In the example above, more of those people would

ANSWERS

have a false positive due to diet/medicine inges-tion, so specificity would go down. The specificity of the Hemoccult II test is 98% when performed under ideal circumstances.

179–D

The majority of advanced colorectal neoplasms occur in the distal colon. Flexible sigmoidoscopy to the splenic flexure will identify most of these. This detection rate would likely increase to 90% if combined with FOBT. The prevalence of proxi-mal disease increases with age.

180–A

Screening for colon cancer is controversial. How-ever, any type of screening after age 50 is prefer-able to no screening at all and all methods of screening have been shown to decrease cancer mortality. At this point in time, all of the follow-ing screening strategies are approved for the average risk patient: annual fecal occult blood testing, flexible sigmoidoscopy every five years, FOBT annually and sigmoidoscopy every five years, double-contrast barium enema every five to 10 years, or colonoscopy every 10 years.

181–C

Mitral valve prolapse (57%) and valvular regurgi-tation (17%) are the most common types of valvu-lar disease in Down syndrome adults. Patients with significant regurgitation or recent cardiac surgery require antibiotic prophylaxis. Careful cardiac auscultation as well as symptom assessment is sufficient to screen for cardiac function.

182–E

Behavioral change is the common presenting pathway of many conditions for adults with Down syndrome. Hearing loss occurs in 70% of patients and may not present until adulthood. Obstructive sleep apnea and hypothyroidism are also very prevalent. Nonspecific complaints should be aggressively pursued in this population.

183–A

In ages 60–69, up to 75% of Down syndrome patients will show symptoms of Alzheimer's. Mood disorders are present in approximately 30% of these same patients. Obsessive-compulsive disorder and autism are more common in Down syndrome patients than in the general population.

184–A

There is a bimodal distribution of onset of seizures in patients with Down syndrome: infancy (most common) and the fourth to fifth decade.

185–C

The patient has alpha-thalassemia trait, characterized by a decreased hemoglobin A2. Alpha-thalassemia trait is caused by deletion of two of the four genes that code for the alpha chain subunit in hemoglobin. The following are the electrophoresis patterns for other thalassemia states:

Beta-thalassemia minor: increased Hb A2, increased Hb F, may have normal Hb A.
Beta-thalassemia major: persistence of Hb F
Alpha-thalassemia silent carrier state: normal Hb A, no clinical manifestations

186–C

Heinz bodies are intracellular inclusions formed by the precipitation of Hb H, when synthesis of the alpha-chain subunits is markedly impaired. Hemoglobin Bart's is a tetramer of gamma chains. Hemoglobin H is a tetramer of beta chains. Hemo-globin Bart's disease is the absence of all four alpha chain genes, and is incompatible with life; hydrops fetalis occurs in utero, because oxygen transport depends on the heterotetramers of either alpha2-beta2 or alpha2-gamma2 in the fetus. The multiple miscarriages for this patient and his wife can be attributed to the likelihood that they both have alpha-thalassemia trait, with resultant offspring having all four alpha-chain gene deletions, yielding hemoglobin Bart's disease.

187–C

Splenomegaly is expected in beta-thalassemia major. Other signs include those of anemia (pallor, tachycardia), chipmunk facies, and hepatomegaly.

188–A

Ferrous sulfate would be contraindicated in a patient with beta-thalassemia major; in fact, prevention and treatment of iron overload is a mainstay of treatment in these patients. This highlights the importance of distinguishing between iron deficiency anemia and thalassemia, rather than empirically treating any microcytic-hypochromic anemia with iron. Splenectomy is indicated in those patients with severe RBC destruction; Pneumovax should be administered to patients who undergo splenectomy. Blood transfusions are used to treat severe anemia, but there is an increased risk for iron overload. Bone marrow transplantation is the definitive treatment for patients with a histocompatible donor.

189–B

Based on Framingham point scores of estimated 10-year risk of MI in men, this patient's risk is 8% for 10 years. This risk data is based on age, total cholesterol, smoking status, HDL, and blood pressure. A 10-year risk greater than 20% is considered equivalent to having coronary artery disease. These tables for men and women can be accessed through the NIH and are the product of the National Cholesterol Education Program, Adult Treatment Program III, 2001.

190–B

New recommendations for cholesterol management base treatment goals on the patient's risk factors as well as the patient's estimated 10-year risk of CAD. This patient has risk factors of HTN and age (men > 45, women > 55) and an intermediate 10-year risk of CAD. Patients with fewer than two risk factors have a goal LDL less than 160; our patient has a goal LDL less than 130. Note: high HDL (over 60) cancels out another risk factor.

191–A

Patients with personal history of coronary artery disease, diabetes, symptomatic carotid artery disease, peripheral arterial disease, abdominal aortic aneurysm, or a 10-year CAD risk of more than 20% should aim for an LDL less than 100. Nephrotic syndrome may itself be a cause of hyperlipidemia, but does not alter the risk of CAD.

192–D

For this patient, who is within 30 mg/dL of his goal, a trial of dietary intervention is certainly reasonable.

TABLE A192. Dietary Intervention

	CHOLESTEROL/ DAY	TOTAL CALORIES FROM FAT	TOTAL CALORIES FROM SATURATED FAT
Step I AHA diet	<300 mg (one egg)	<30%	<10%
Step II AHA diet	<200 mg	<30%, May address fat subtype	<7%

Pharmacologic therapy could also be considered. The role of red wine in coronary artery disease is still debated; this patient's lipid profile would not be helped by adding more wine to his one to two glasses per night. Alcohol ingestion increases triglycerides transiently; in greater amounts it can cause hyperlipidemia.

193–D

Onset of levothyroxine is gradual; it can take up to six weeks for a dose to become fully effective. TSH is a more physiologic reflection than FT4 of the thyroid state of the body; it is also much more sensitive because it correlates by inverse logarithm to the circulating thyroid hormone. (Therefore a drop in FT4 by 60%—still a normal value—would trigger an almost threefold increase in TSH—clearly abnormal.) TSH can take even longer than eight weeks to reflect the physiologic state, so the patient's symptoms should also be assessed before increasing the levothyroxine dose for a still elevated TSH. FT4 need only be checked if the TSH has increased or if it is very low (less than 0.1).

194–B

Hypothyroidism is a secondary cause of hyperlipidemia (increased LDL and lowered HDL), due to decreased catabolism of VLDL and IDL. Hyperthyroidism would correct this. Inducing a hyperthyroid state can cause all of the symptoms of primary hyperthyroidism including osteoporosis, exacerbation of CAD, arrhythmias, and anxiety.

195–D

By definition, this patient has subclinical hypothyroidism: TSH between 5 and 10 mU/L in an asymptomatic patient. (The TSH had been ordered as a screening test; therefore, she was asymptomatic.) Management is somewhat controversial. About 20% of patients with subclinical hypothyroidism will develop overt hypothyroidism within five years. Patients with high titers of antithyroid antibodies are at highest risk. No randomized, controlled studies have shown benefit to treatment with levothyroxine of a TSH between 5 and 10. Early treatment does not prevent progression. Approaches vary as to the management; some clinicians would check a FT4 immediately with antithyroid antibodies, and possibly treat if positive for antibodies. Others would retest the TSH in six months to a year unless the patient developed symptoms.

ANSWERS

196–A

There are many different recommendations for thyroid function test screening at the present time. There is a general consensus to consider mass screening for thyroid dysfunction in women over the age of 60, but the U.S. Preventive Task Force guidelines do not fully endorse that currently.

197–D

Hemoglobin A1C should be measured every three to six months depending on the tightness of control desired. In addition to the other tests, lipids should be measured and controlled annually, and smoking status should be addressed and counseled.

198–A

Hyperglycemia leads to poor white-cell functioning and is considered an immunocompromised state. Influenza and pneumonia cause significant morbidity and mortality in diabetics.

199–B

Type 2 DM usually progresses over time as the pancreas "burns out" or is able to produce less and less insulin for the insulin-resistant body—use of exogenous insulin therapy increases as the disease progresses. Mortality from diabetes is weighted: 60-75% of people with diabetes die from cardiovascular causes. This great risk has led to more intensive recommendations for primary (before known cardiac disease) and secondary (after known cardiac disease) prevention of CV morbidity in diabetics. These recommendations include: aspirin as primary and secondary prevention, aggressive lipid control, tight BP control, and CABG over PTCA for multivessel disease.

200–B

TCAs have been well-studied for this indication. They are inexpensive and have a good number needed to treat of approximately 3.0 (need to treat three patients for one to feel significant improvement). Their side-effect profile, which includes sedation, urinary retention, and constipation, is much less problematic at the doses used for neuropathy than in the higher doses required to treat depression. Gabapentin is likely as efficacious with fewer side effects, but is much more costly and has no long-term studies. Mexilitine has no good evidence and carbamazepine causes too many side effects.

132

INDEX

INDEX